The Palgrave Lacan Series

Jacques Lacan is one of the most important and influential thinkers of the 20th century. The reach of this influence continues to grow as we settle into the 21st century, the resonance of Lacan's thought arguably only beginning now to be properly felt, both in terms of its application to clinical matters and in its application to a range of human activities and interests. The Palgrave Lacan Series is a book series for the best new writing in the Lacanian field, giving voice to the leading writers of a new generation of Lacanian thought. The series will comprise original monographs and thematic, multi-authored collections. The books in the series will explore aspects of Lacan's theory from new perspectives and with original insights. There will be books focused on particular areas of or issues in clinical work. There will be books focused on applying Lacanian theory to areas and issues beyond the clinic, to matters of society, politics, the arts and culture. Each book, whatever its particular concern, will work to expand our understanding of Lacan's theory and its value in the 21st century.

More information about this series at
http://www.palgrave.com/gp/series/15116

Bret Fimiani

Psychosis and Extreme States

An Ethic for Treatment

palgrave
macmillan

Bret Fimiani
The San Francisco Bay Area Lacanian School of Psychoanalysis
Berkeley, CA, USA

The Palgrave Lacan Series
ISBN 978-3-030-75439-6 ISBN 978-3-030-75440-2 (eBook)
https://doi.org/10.1007/978-3-030-75440-2

This Palgrave Macmillan imprint is published by the registered company Springer Nature Switzerland AG.
The registered company address is: Gewerbestrasse 11, 6330 Cham, Switzerland

for Hailey

Foreword

Once, on a long walk towards a downtown restaurant for dinner, as we tacked through the streets and hills of San Francisco, Bret brought me to see the place where he worked. Approaching Tenderloin Health Services we dodged pigeons and blinked in the strong light that cut the shadows of tall buildings into intricate geometries. Bret greeted people on the street. We took an elevator ride and walked through a layer of offices and waiting rooms. Bret greeted people with ease, introducing me as he went. I could readily imagine him in his office with someone seeking words for disarray and strangeness, and Bret making a place for the lived experience of psychosis with characteristic respect and calm. We'd met nearly two decades previously in seminars on psychoanalysis offered in Quebec City. Now we were both analysts of the Bay Area Lacanian School of Psychoanalysis. We had each been interested in the treatment of psychosis for many years, Bret through his training as an analyst and his clinical work, and I as a writer, analyst, and one who had experienced psychosis repeatedly in my youth.

When Bret asked me to write this foreword, I answered in the affirmative right away, knowing that he had been immersed in questions about clinical work with psychosis for many years, as long as I'd known him. I'd read his doctoral thesis during our Quebec years, a rigorous exploration of dreams in the treatment of psychosis. As I waited to get his manuscript in the mail, I wondered what he would say about psychosis now. I opened the package of his chapters and began to read. The chapter titles alone intrigued me. Introducing his book with "The Psychotic as Guide", Bret's writing, I could see immediately, drew from his incisive questions, his layered readings of Lacan and beyond Lacan, and his detailed renderings from the clinic of his practice. He seemed to be orienting his readers with a compass whose north star was the experience of psychosis, and its directions the body, knowledge, and ethics of the psychotic as subject.

While the "medical world" is interested primarily in eliminating psychotic symptoms, and many doctors as well as other professionals appear frightened of the strangeness of psychosis, Bret's book shows us a way to actually listen to psychotic speech. Listening well makes it possible to move beyond fear, to build a credible address for people experiencing psychosis, and to discover a way to accompany them into a new trajectory of hope.

Drawing on the clinic, philosophy, psychoanalysis, the Hearing Voices Network, and his extensive interviews with colleagues working in the area of psychosis (including with me), Bret questions orthodoxies and received knowledge (in psychiatry, psychology, and psychoanalysis) to forge a creative, ethical, and courageous treatment of psychosis. It is a book that is very much needed in our time, needed in the way of a deep drink of cold well water after a long time of thirst, needed as if one were dying of thirst in fact, and had been offered some tepid, poisoned liquid in lieu of water for years. It is a guide for clinicians, especially for analysts, but also for anyone interested in psychosis as a singular, enigmatic, terrifying experience, an experience sometimes beyond words.

Amherst, MA

Annie G. Rogers

Acknowledgements

I would first like to thank several friends/colleagues/mentors who read drafts of the manuscript and who provided me with encouragement and editorial suggestions when I needed them the most. Thank you to Juliet Flower MacCannell for her generosity in initially reading select chapters and then the entire manuscript. Juliet's insightful feedback was invaluable and her encouragement arrived just in time and helped me very much to move forward at a critical point in the writing process. Annie Rogers gave much to this project and I am grateful to her for her numerous contributions to this book. First, I knew in advance that Annie would be the perfect person to write the foreword and her beautifully written contribution far exceeded my already very high expectations. Annie's responses in the course of her interview in Chap. 8 were illuminating and a vital part of this book. Finally, Annie also generously served as a reader and her feedback and editorial advice were indispensable to the completion of the book. Françoise Davoine was very supportive of this project and I am grateful to her for her groundbreaking work in the field of psychosis. Davoine and Jean-Max Gaudilliere's work in *History Beyond Trauma* has inspired my most recent thinking on ethics and psychosis. Françoise also generously served as a reader and provided much needed encouragement and valuable editorial advice. I interviewed Barri Belnap on the topic of the 'fear of psychosis' for this project and I thank her for her keen insights, and for her openness and honesty in discussing this difficult and important topic. Barri's work in the field of psychosis is inspiring.

There are many clinicians and writers whose work on psychosis has inspired me and lighted the way on this path to better understand, and be of use to, people with extreme experiences. However, there are a few key people I would like to thank in particular. My early training in the psychoanalysis of psychosis was via the training seminars taught by the founding analysts of GIFRIC. Their important work with psychosis really should be better known. In particular, case consultation with Lucie Cantin, nearly 20 years ago, was pivotal in my learning to truly listen to psychosis. I thank my close friend and colleague of over 20 years, Christopher Meyer, for the countless energizing and insight-producing conversations about psychoanalysis and psychosis that have helped motivate and guide me along the way.

Thank you to the Bay Area Hearing Voices Network (BAHVN) for their extremely important work with people who experience voice hearing, unusual beliefs, and other extraordinary perceptions. I am grateful to be a BAHVN board member and to have the privilege to learn about recovery from people with lived experience. My understanding of 'psychosis' and my clinical practice has been forever changed for the better by my opportunity to collaborate with the Hearing Voices Network (HVN). I have devoted an entire chapter to the findings of the HVN and its relevance to the understanding and treatment of psychosis. I thank HVN member and educator Cindy Marty Hadge for allowing me to interview her for this book. Cindy's moving testimony about her own recovery, her powerful insights into the problems with our mental health system, and her guidance on how best to listen to other voice hearers are essential contributions to this book.

I thank my publisher Palgrave Macmillan for the opportunity to publish this work and I thank the editorial and production staff for their support in bringing this project to completion. In particular I thank Derrick Hook for his support and for welcoming me to add my work to the Palgrave Lacan Book Series.

I thank my parents Sally and Mike Wiley for all of their support and encouragement.

Finally, I thank my wife Hailey and our sons August and Miles for their support during the completion of this book. Hailey knew that I could write this book before I did. I wrote a large part of this book during the 2020–2021 Covid-19 pandemic and, like so many others, my family and I were living in close quarters around the clock, overseeing distance learning, and carrying out our professional responsibilities all under one roof. I thank my family for making adjustments to their own routines to allow me the space and time to write, for their enthusiasm for this project, and for showing me constant encouragement during the writing process.

Contents

About the Author

Dr. Bret Fimiani is a psychoanalyst of the San Francisco Bay Area Lacanian School of Psychoanalysis. He is also a clinical psychologist. He works with people experiencing psychosis and extreme states in his private practice in Oakland, CA, and at the Haight-Ashbury Integrated Care Center in San Francisco. He is the chairperson for the Northern California Chapter of the International Society for the Psychological and Social Approaches to Psychosis and he is on the board of directors for the Bay Area Hearing Voices Network. His research interests include adapting the Lacanian analytic framework for the treatment of psychosis and extreme states, and the integration of peer and clinical models. He has presented his work on the treatment of psychosis nationally and internationally.

List of Figures

1

Introduction: The Psychotic as Guide

The goal of this project is to move towards a theory of transference-in-psychosis that will provoke a change in the way the experience of psychosis is understood and, thus, clinically treated. My specific question is with regard to the function of 'ethics'[1] in the 'installation' of transference in the treatment of psychosis. In my approach, the problem of the installation of transference raises the question of ethics because, I contend, the aim of the psychoanalytic experience is the creation of a new ethic for the analysand. I see the psychotic's 'choice' to enter transference (redefined as a 'desire to know') as linked to the creation of a new ethic—in which 'ethics' concerns the emergence of a new 'responsibility' on the part of the psychotic. Furthermore, I suggest that it is through an account of the specific knowledge (*savoir*) implicit in the psychotic experience that psychoanalysis can maintain its bearings as an 'ethical praxis'.

Basing my approach on the work of psychoanalyst Jacques Lacan and philosopher Gilles Deleuze (regarding the body in particular), I begin

[1] My thesis regarding 'ethics in psychosis' follows, in a particular way, Jacques Lacan's exploration of the problem of ethics (1993) in psychoanalysis in *The Seminar of Jacques Lacan, Book VII The Ethics of Psychoanalysis 1959–1960*. I provide a brief initial elaboration of the term "ethics" (and its clinical implications) in this Introduction. I fully define and elaborate the question of 'ethics' in Chap. 6.

B. Fimiani, *Psychosis and Extreme States*, The Palgrave Lacan Series,
https://doi.org/10.1007/978-3-030-75440-2_1

with the premise that the body of the psychotic is a site of social contestation. In this framework, the 'organism' is defined as the object of medical science, and biological psychiatry, while the 'body', eroticized by language, is the primary concern of psychoanalysis. This body is the result of a radical disruption (by language and cultural demands) of the original instinctual functioning of the organism. Beginning with this premise, I then suggest that we will be better positioned to guide the psychotic towards a psychoanalytic cure if we first formulate the psychotic's condition as a failed attempt to resist (contest) capture by the demands of social–symbolic exchange and libidinal–economic imperatives.

Drawing upon the work of Freud, Lacan, Deleuze and Guattari, and Apollon et al., this book reframes the problem of the 'body' (as an effect of language) and its relation to transference, and ethics, in treating psychosis. In the course of my research I have found no studies conducted in the North American context that specifically address the problem of the 'body' and transference in psychosis from the perspectives of Freud, Lacan, Deleuze, and Guattari.

It is important for my readers to understand that I distinguish the 'structure' of the psychotic experience from the 'phenomenology' (symptoms) of psychosis. Now, the dominant approaches to treating psychosis in North America derive from the medical/psychiatric model that defines psychosis by reference to a biologically driven understanding of the phenomenology of psychosis. Likewise, contemporary American psychoanalytic approaches have little to say regarding the structure versus the phenomenology of psychosis. The consequence of their common failure to account for structure is that the psychotic experience has continued to be understood as a malfunction of the biological organism and/or a deviation from neurotic-level psychical functioning. In either case, the psychotic experience is reduced to a problem *internal* to the individual (organism or psyche).

To avoid falling into the trap of the 'nature/culture' binarism ("organism/psyche") therefore requires an epistemological critique that undermines the nature/culture binarism itself. Such a critique is implicit in my approach to the theorization of the psychotic experience. For if, as I suggest, the 'body of the psychotic' is a contestation of the fundament of the symbolic universe, then the structure of knowledge itself is called into question, including the knowledge(s), or discourses, that have attempted historically to take the psychotic experience as their 'object' (e.g., medical science/psychiatry, and psychoanalysis). To suppose a 'subject' of the psychotic experience is to suppose a specific knowledge of the psychotic that calls all general and expert knowledge(s) into question.

1.1 From the Body to Ethics

My hypothesis is that the phenomenon of contestation manifest in psychosis is key to the development of an ethics in the analytic experience—the ethics of both the analyst and analysand. 'Ethics' is here understood as situating the psychotic subject in relation to a failed Law and to death drive.

In this book, I am not using the term ethics in the sense understood by North American practitioners in psychology or psychiatry as the 'code of professional ethics'. Rather, I theorize the question of 'ethics' by extracting the true stakes of Kant's moral Law (categorical imperative) by reading Kant after Lacan and in light of the psychotic's *savoir*. The problem is that of constructing an 'ethics without ethics'—in other words, an ethics without the guarantee of Aristotle's Good or Kant's "moral law within". Ultimately, this way of understanding ethics directly affects the clinic and potentially bears consequences for our conception of ethics in the social sphere as well.

Positing the body of the psychotic as a site of social contestation further requires a re-theorization of the body itself. One theoretical concern of this study is to challenge biological determinist readings of Freud's drive theory.[2] Maintenance of the distinction between 'drive' and 'instinct' allows for an understanding of a second body—the body of drive (versus instinct). I contend that the re-theorization of the body requires a return

[2] The translation of Freud's '*trieb*' as 'instinct' is fundamental to the misunderstanding of drive theory as biologically based. Laplanche and Pontalis (1973), in The Language of Psychoanalysis, state that, in the case of the English-speaking psychoanalytic community, "[t]he word 'instinct' is used to translate two different German words, '*Instinkt*' and '*Trieb*'" (214). An important conceptual difference is lost in this act of translation. The effect of collapsing the conceptual distinction between instinct and drive is to produce a concept of the body as either on or off an 'instinctual track'.

to Freud in order to articulate a drive theory of psychosis which, however, necessitates a passage through the re-readings of Freud by Lacan and Deleuze and Guattari. They offer a novel way to read Freud and to understand the true status of drive (versus instinct), i.e., to consider drive as the effect of language. More precisely, as in Chap. 1 where I discuss the 'body' as an effect of the trauma of Language on the 'organism': drive is to the 'body' as instinct is to the 'organism'. The crucial point is that the psychotic's unique relation to Language is fundamentally 'traumatic'.

In psychosis, we have a specific type of social contestation that is the result of a forced choice and therefore a choice prior to the entrance into the transference, and thus prior to the creation of an ethic. In *Seminar III, The Psychoses* (1992), Lacan theorized that the psychotic psychical structure is determined by a radical exclusion ("foreclosure") of the primary word or "signifier" that, for neurotic subjects, comes to provide a first link in the subject's effort to make sense of experience. Thus the psychotic is without the primary, or fundamental, (symbolic) link to anchor the structure of psychical reality: and the 'body', as defined in this book, is a 'psychical reality'.

I argue that "foreclosure" is the result of the psychotic's (first) 'choice' in life: a choice deployed at the moment of the 'advent of the subject'. The psychotic's 'first choice' is to radically exclude ("foreclose") the symbolic anchoring point for Sense and meaning. I argue that situating the psychotic's "foreclosure" as a 'choice' is in fact the precondition for psychoanalysis and, by extension, the precondition for a new 'freedom' for the psychotic subject. However, this first 'choice' bears certain disastrous consequences for the psychotic: without the anchoring point for Sense, she retreats into the closed universe of delusion and the 'violence' of the persecutory voices.

Yet it is of particular importance here to note that the psychotic's 'choice' of foreclosure also yields a specific 'knowledge' (*savoir*) regarding the foundation of the 'Law' and the Ideals that support the rules of social coexistence. It is the psychotic's *savoir* of the Law that guides us in defining and theorizing an ethics and, furthermore, in formulating the aim of analysis as creating the conditions for a 'second' (ethical) choice in the face of the effects of the Law that return when the delusion is ruptured. I argue that the psychotic's entrance into transference, defined as a desire to know, constitutes a 'second' choice to enter the field of ethics and thus to assume a new 'responsibility for death drive'.

Thus to make contact with the 'subject of psychosis' we must begin with the body of the drive, where the psychotic (in her disorganized body) finds herself stranded without speech and without the fundamental word necessary to begin the articulation of her experience. The psychotic, if given the place to speak, will reveal her subjective truth as well as the truth of the Law itself.

My thesis, then, is that there is a correspondence between the psychotic's *savoir* and the truth (or 'principle') behind the moral Law. The psychotic's *savoir* of the Law will take us further than even Lacan's powerful critique of Kantian ethics. The objective here is twofold: we aim to gain a clarified understanding of the moral Law itself, which, in turn, allows the analyst to better understand the symbolic (i.e., ethical) position required to invite the psychotic into the transference defined as a desire-to-know. The psychotic will not respond, except with "indifference" or paranoia, to anything other than the analyst's genuine desire 'to know' the truth of the psychotic's experience. Whereas Lacan based his interrogation of traditional ethics upon the neurotic's libidinal 'tie', we will allow the psychotic to lead the inquiry. *An understanding of the psychotic's experience, and specific knowledge, of the moral Law is fundamental to an effective treatment of psychosis.*

1.2 Ethics and the Clinic

The aim of the psychoanalytic experience is the construction of a new ethic for the subject. I deploy the term 'ethics' to capture and explain the subjective shift that may occur in the course of treatment wherein the subject of psychosis assumes a level of responsibility for her experience—hence my question regarding the function of 'choice' in the experience, and in the treatment of psychosis. The said 'shift' implies that the psychotic (in the course of treatment) moves from the position of 'object' to that of the 'subject'.

In addition, my usage of the term 'ethics' regards the nature of the subject's position in relation to the failure of the pleasure principle

(Biology) and to the unfoundedness of symbolic castration (or Law). The term 'ethics' therefore refers to a particular subject's specific way of facing death drive, insofar as death drive (or "jouissance")[3] is that which is 'beyond the pleasure principle' and in 'excess' of any symbolic limit. Psychoanalyst Willy Apollon (2002) writes:

> The Lacanian clinic favors an ethics where *savoir* [specific knowledge] is substituted for a *jouissance* that the treatment experience reveals as lapsed and thus impossible. (After Lacan, p. 140)

Apollon's remark implies that, through the analytic experience, the analysand constructs a new knowledge (*savoir*) that creates the conditions for an ethical choice: the subject can choose the symptom (addiction, obsession, delusion) or face what Apollon calls the necessary "failure of *jouissance*" (p. 140). Apollon's reference to "failure" speaks to the interface between Language and the organism, and between the Law, castration, and drive, a linkage elaborated throughout this book. It will suffice here to remark that the "failure of jouissance" is a requirement for the subject of desire to emerge, and to construct an ethics based upon the stakes of desire and lack, insofar as desire *is* a 'failure' or a lack introduced into the fullness of an imagined satisfaction (jouissance). However, I argue that, given the psychotic's "foreclosure" of the Name-of-the-Father and its consequences, the installation of transference in the field of psychosis marks the introduction of 'desire itself': thus the stakes for the psychotic (versus the neurotic) are necessarily higher.

With respect to the clinic, the problem of ethics is particularly relevant to my question regarding the problematic of the psychotic's entrance into transference: a question that stems from the linkage between

[3] " Jouissance" translates roughly as enjoyment, but jouissance is not simply pleasure. Jouissance is a complex term that evolves over the course of Lacan's body of work. For this study I will situate jouissance in the category of what is impossible for the human, namely total satisfaction (e.g., the object of "instinctual renunciation"). However, in the clinical context suggested by Apollon (following Lacan), the term jouissance also implies pleasure, but a pleasure that is overwhelming and painful, precisely because the pleasure (a quantity of energy) exceeds a certain limit (e.g., a prohibition). As noted in the introduction to *After Lacan* (2002), "*Jouissance* is tied to pleasure, but only the sort of pleasure for which one would suffer endless pain" (p. 29). I have argued elsewhere (2001) that in severe cases of addiction we have an example of a social practice (or social 'symptom') in which an individual is willing to risk his life to gain access to 'total satisfaction' or jouissance.

'contestation, ethics and the transference'. This question is 'what precisely causes the psychotic to enter the transference?' My hypothesis is that the 'cause' is itself dialectical in nature insofar as the "desire of the analyst" (as both 'cause' and 'support') is in play in the provocation of the transference. Is the movement into the transference (for the psychotic) a choice based upon a new ethics vis-à-vis the 'trauma of language'? A 'second' choice, and an ethics, after the 'trauma'?

The following questions guide the discussion of clinical material in Chap. 6, and hopefully provide the reader with a sense of the stakes of this project:

1. What is the ethic of the analyst: on what does the analyst base their action and 'justify' their offering to the psychotic?
2. How can we locate the dream as a "psychoanalytic dream" that, by definition, calls the certainty of delusion into question?
3. Where, in treatment, does the subject of the unconscious appear in the dream-work to challenge/contest the certainty of delusion and the command of the Voice?
4. How does the patient respond to the contestation of delusion by the work of the dream, and the appearance of the subject?
5. Did a new ethic emerge on the side of the patient? In other words, did the patient choose to put a new *savoir* (a lacking knowledge) in place of certainty?
6. Finally, how do we theorize the presence or absence of a shift towards an ethical position for the subject of psychosis?

The theoretical inquiry into the questions of the body, transference, the dream, and ethics is fundamental to our effort to answer these questions.

1.3 The Fear of Psychosis

The latter chapters of this book will address the topic of the 'fear of psychosis' based upon a set of diverse perspectives. I contend that there is a powerful fear of psychosis (and of "madness") that pervades our healthcare system, including within the disciplines of psychology, psychiatry, and psychoanalysis. The fear of psychosis leads to treatment approaches that are reductive, sometimes harsh, and stigmatizing. First, I will explore the topic of fear via the perspective of people with lived experience of psychosis. People with lived experience of psychosis offer new insights into (1) the experience of being the object of fear-based approaches to treatment and, by contrast, (2) the healing experience of encountering a respectful and curious listener. Furthermore, in contrast to fear-based clinical approaches, I will explore the vital importance of a peer-driven approach to psychosis, namely the Hearing Voices Network (HVN). HVN is a peer-facilitated group-based approach to living with psychosis that was founded by people with lived experience of psychosis. Towards the goal of learning from people with lived experience of psychosis, I have included an interview with a member and educator within the HVN. In my assessment, HVN has spontaneously discovered methods to "treat"[4] the experience of distress that can so often accompany voice hearing and distressing beliefs (i.e., delusions). Furthermore, HVN's perspective and practices have much to teach clinicians regarding how best to position oneself *ethically* in order to connect with people experiencing psychosis.

Second, I will explore the topic of 'fear' from a clinical perspective via interviews with practitioners of psychoanalysis and psychiatry. The insights that follow from these interviews, in addition to my analysis of the theoretical and clinical work of psychoanalysts Françoise Davione and Jean-Max Gaudilliere, will illuminate how the fear of psychosis can lead to transference impasses.

[4] I am aware that the term 'treat', or 'treatment', is at odds with the principles and the Charter of the Hearing Voices Network (HVN). The term 'treatment', as defined within the medical model, directly implies that psychosis, and in particular voice hearing, is an 'illness'. The HVN Charter states that voice hearing, within the HVN approach, is not considered a sign of illness per se. HVN is careful to avoid terms that, historically, issue from the medical model and that therefore pathologize and often stigmatize the experience of psychosis. In Chap. 7, I will address and explain my decision to use (reclaim) the term 'treatment' with regard to the HVN and its methods. In short, and by contrast, my use of the term 'treatment' within the framework of psychoanalysis is also at odds with the way the term is deployed within the medical model. Both my psychoanalytic approach and the HVN approach operate outside the medical model and, I argue, strive to dignify the experience of psychosis rather than relegate it to being purely an illness. See my commentary section in Chap. 7 that follows the interview with peer-specialist and educator Cindy Marty Hadge for an elaboration of my approach to reappropriating the term 'treatment'.

This book is divided into nine chapters: (1) "Introduction: The Psychotic as Guide", (2) "The Body of the Psychotic", (3) "The Impasse of Transference in Psychosis", (4) "The Dream-work Versus Delusion", (5) "The Utility of Gilles Deleuze's Critique of Psychoanalysis", (6) "Towards a New Ethics", (7) "The Fear of psychosis: Part I", (8) "The Fear of psychosis: Part II", and (9) "Bridging the Gap Between Psychotic and Non-Psychotic Experience".

In Chap. 1, I provide the rationale for the book and an overview of the structure of the book, including chapter summaries. In brief, I articulate how my reformulations of the body of psychosis, transference, dream-work, and ethics are key for a psychoanalytic approach in the clinic of psychosis. In addition I summarize my argument for an inclusion, within psychoanalysis, of the perspectives of people with lived experience of psychosis and, in particular, the importance of the Hearing Voices Network/Movement for both psychosis and psychoanalysis. Finally, I present my assessment of the shortcomings of the orthodox Lacanian notion of analytic neutrality when working clinically with psychosis.

In Chap. 2, I present my theorization of the 'body of the psychotic' from a Freudian–Lacanian psychoanalytic (versus medical) perspective. I offer a reading of Freud's *Project for a Scientific Psychology* (1895), *Three Essays on Sexuality* (1905), *Instincts and their Vicissitudes* (1915), and *Beyond the Pleasure Principle* (1920) to render what in his text problematizes biological determinist interpretations of his theory of the 'instincts'. In the *Project*, a "pre-psychoanalytic" text, Freud is on his way to discovering the true stakes, for the subject, of the primary loss of the 'object' of satisfaction, and the way in which the "first registration" (a *Niederschriften* or "writing down") of the 'first loss' in turn creates the 'body'. We will follow Freud and Lacan in order to locate the contours of the psychotic's first encounter with Language and to begin to theorize the psychotic's experience of the "first registration" of loss. I argue that what is at stake for the psychotic is the lack of any 'justification' for loss, insofar as the Name-of the-Father (or primary representation) functions for the neurotic to repress the 'unjustifiable' status of loss itself.

In Chap. 3, I suggest a way to re-conceptualize the transference that follows from the new understanding of the body of the psychotic, as well as from the consequences of the psychotic's "foreclosure." The main task of Chap. 3 is to isolate the stakes of the 'transference-impasse' reached by both Freud and Lacan and, thus, to open the way for a redefinition of transference that will serve the psychotic.

In Chap. 4, I theorize the structural difference between the dream and delusion, and suggest a way to 'treat' delusion via the symbolic work of the dream. Here, I redefine transference strictly in terms of 'knowledge': transference defined as a 'desire for unconscious knowledge'. Ultimately, I argue that for the analyst to enter the psychotic experience requires a "reversal" of transference, thus modifying the usual analytic positions. In this chapter I also use clinical examples to ground the theorization of the function of the dream versus delusion.

Chapter 5 serves as a preliminary to the discussion of 'ethics', which is the substance of Chap. 6. In this chapter I address Deleuze's claim that psychoanalysis "botches the encounter with the psychotic", and then demonstrate that Deleuze's concept of the "Body without Organs" is key to understanding what is at stake in the psychotic's experience.

In Chap. 6, I show that the "reversal", and therefore the installation, of transference depends upon the isolation of the field of ethics: an 'ethics derived from the psychotic's singular knowledge (*savoir*) of the moral Law'. Under transference, defined as a 'desire to know', the psychotic's delusion (as solution and defence) will 'fall' and thus expose the psychotic to the Void of both language and the moral Law. By what means, or 'term', can the psychotic bear the Law and its Void? This book proposes that the fall ('rupture') of delusion opens the 'field' of ethics, and thus marks the threshold the psychotic must cross to inaugurate her journey towards becoming a desiring subject. I argue that the task is to locate the field and function of ethics in the context of the experience and treatment of psychosis.

In Chap. 7, I address the topic of the 'fear of psychosis'. In doing so, I expand the scope of approaches to psychosis to include the perspective of people with lived experience of psychosis and I explore the importance of a peer-driven model, namely the Hearing Voices Network (HVN). Ultimately, I argue that the HVN and my psychoanalytic model share a 'common ethical stance' and both approaches understand delusions and the content of voices as forms of knowledge. My interview with peer-specialist and educator Cindy Marty Hadge, as well as my conceptual discussion that follows the interview, will illuminate the stakes and consequences of the 'common ethic'.

In Chap. 8, I extend the discussion of the 'fear of psychosis'. The discussion, both clinical and conceptual, again revolves around interviews with people particularly well suited to provide new insights into the problem of fear. From the dual perspective of a person with lived experience of psychosis and that of psychoanalyst and scholar, Dr. Annie Rogers helps us understand how the curiosity (versus fearfulness) of the analyst creates a space for the person with psychosis to speak openly while also feeling safe from judgement, misunderstanding, and stigma. My discussion with Dr. Rogers also opens up an important discussion of the various versions of the 'Other' that can populate the experience of psychosis, e.g., the Other as destroyed, capricious, or enigmatic, or the "Other as a far-horizon". My discussion with psychiatrist and psychoanalyst Dr. Barri Belnap illuminates how affording psychotic experience a certain "dignity" in the process of mutual understanding can effectively combat the corrosive effect of fear and the impulse to 'control' that so often follows from fearfulness. Dr. Belnap also provides important insights into the precarious nature and status of 'authority' for, in particular, someone living with psychosis.

In Chap. 9, I revisit the problematic of transference, and traditional Lacanian notions of the analytic relation, with regard to psychosis. More specifically, I explore the possibility of a "shared truth" between the analyst and the person experiencing psychosis. Are there moments with particular patients when the analyst may be called upon to reveal their own relation to the failure of words to account for loss and trauma? This question sets up a confrontation between the well-known dictate, and position, of analytic neutrality and an alternative position where the analyst may be called upon to explicitly acknowledge how trauma is created via the "annulment" of loss. 'Annulment' renders loss non-existent, thus creating a hole or "zone of death" in one's experience. I understand zones of death, or zones of "non-existence", to be common to the human experience (i.e., universal). Thus, I suggest, in revealing his or her encounter with 'annulment' and erasure, the analyst is speaking about (and to) the universal strangeness of encountering loss-without-words. As noted earlier, the theoretical and clinical work of Françoise Davoine and Jean-Max

Gaudilliere will serve as a guide in understanding how we can traverse such "zones of death/non-existence" in order to bridge the gap between psychotic and non-psychotic experience. My discussion of how to enter and inhabit shared zones of non-existence will open the way to approach the challenge of "co-creating a credible address" for the treatment of psychosis.

References

Apollon, W. (2002). From symptom to fantasy. In R. Hughes & K. R. Malone (Eds.), *After Lacan: Clinical practice and the subject of the unconscious* (pp. 127–140). SUNY Press.

Freud, S. (1895). *Project for a scientific psychology*. In J. Strachey (Ed. and Trans.), *The standard edition of the complete psychological works od Sigmund Freud* (Vol. I, pp. 283–397). Hogarth Press, 1999.

Freud, S. (1905). *Three essays on sexuality*. SE Vol. VII, 1999, pp. 135–243.

Freud, S. (1915). Instincts and their vicissitudes. SE Vol. XIV, 1999, pp. 114–140.

Freud, S. (1920). *Beyond the pleasure principle*. SE XVIII: 1999, pp. 3–63.

Lacan, J. (1992). *The ethics of psychoanalysis (1959–1960), The seminar of Jacques Lacan, Book VII* (J.A. Miller, Ed., and D. Porter, Trans.). W.W. Norton & Co.

Lacan, J. (1993). *The psychoses (1955–1956), The seminar of Jacques Lacan, Book III* (J.A. Miller, Ed., and R. Grigg, Trans.). W.W. Norton & Co.

Laplanche, J., & Pontalis, J. B. (1973). *The language of psychoanalysis*. W.W. Norton & Co.

2

The Body of the Psychotic

2.1 The 'Unjustifiable' Status of Loss

To move towards an analysis of the stakes of transference in psychosis first requires the construction of a unique understanding of the body of the psychotic. The body, as opposed to the organism, is the result of a radical disruption by Language and cultural demands of the instinctual functioning of the organism. The disruption of the organism implies the mapping of drive over instinct and the introduction of an unconscious logic of the body in opposition to the bio-logic of the organism. Fundamentally, the said rupture of instinctual functioning—the rupture of the organism—implies a radical loss of satisfaction. Three main questions guide our inquiry regarding the unique stakes, for the psychotic, of a radical loss of satisfaction: (1) What is the psychotic's specific relation to the failure of biological and symbolic limits? (2) Why is the fundamental, and necessary, loss of satisfaction unbearable for the psychotic versus the neurotic? (3) How does the psychotic's unique relation to the failure

B. Fimiani, *Psychosis and Extreme States*, The Palgrave Lacan Series,
https://doi.org/10.1007/978-3-030-75440-2_2

of symbolic limits (Language) change our understanding of the phenomenology of psychosis? Freud and Lacan will be our guides in answering these questions. I argue that the phenomenology of psychosis must be understood *structurally*. Here structure implies that psychotic phenomena correspond to a defect, or failure, in the structure of Language itself.

In this chapter I offer a reading of Freud's *Project for a Scientific Psychology* (1895), *Three Essays on Sexuality* (1905), *Instincts and their Vicissitudes* (1915a), and *Beyond the Pleasure Principle* (1920) to render what in his text itself problematizes biological determinist interpretations of his theory of the instincts. We will meet Freud where he discovers the failure of any "biological contrivance" or "communication" (speech) to satisfy the constant pressure of "somatic" need. Freud discovers that, given the failure of the "pleasure principle" (for Freud a biological limit), the human has recourse only to symbolic means to find a limit to the suffering introduced by the impossibility of obtaining total satisfaction. In the *Project*, a "pre-psychoanalytic" text, Freud is on his way to discovering the true stakes, for the subject, of the primary loss of the 'object' of satisfaction, and the way in which the "first registration" (a *Niederschriften* or "writing down") of the first loss in turn creates the body.

The primary loss of satisfaction and its consequence (death drive and the body) are facts of experience for every subject whether psychotic, neurotic, or perverse, but the psychotic makes a particular choice in the face of this primary loss of satisfaction: the choice to "foreclose" the Name-of-the-Father. On this point we will follow Freud further in the *Project*, and Lacan in *Seminar III*, in order to locate the contours of the psychotic's first encounter with Language and to begin to theorize the psychotic's experience of the "first registration" of loss. I argue that what is at stake for the psychotic is the lack of any *justification* for loss, insofar as the Name-of the-Father functions for the neurotic to repress the unjustifiable status of loss itself.

2.2 Freud's Discovery of the Body as the Effect of the Lost Object of Satisfaction

Freud is often misunderstood to have constructed a biological determinist theory in which the human being is compelled by instinctual forces.[1] Freud's discovery of the body of drive—a body that lives beyond biology—bears consequences for our understanding of the structure of psychosis, that is, psychosis is a psychical structure oriented by the object of a lost satisfaction or jouissance.

How does Freud theoretically situate the body beyond a certain limit, e.g., the limits of the pleasure principle and symbolic castration? And why, in turn, will highlighting this aspect of Freud's discovery require a new consideration of transference, and ethics, in the experience and clinical treatment of psychosis? The analyst wants to hear from the part of the organism that has been lost. And, what has been lost—as a result of the disorganizing effect of Language—will remain silent, a silence that nonetheless composes the body.

2.2.1 "Quantity" and "quality"

In the *Project for a Scientific Psychology* (1895), Freud initiates a work that opens a space for psychical reality and, I would argue, a place in the discourse of "scientific" psychology for the body. Freud articulates the mode by which the human subject approaches satisfaction via hallucination ("wishful fantasy")—insofar as the object of satisfaction for the human is always an object that merely approximates or aims at satisfaction. In this inquiry Freud discovers that, for the human, the fundamental relation is

[1] Regarding the problem of translation, James Strachey provides a commentary in the general introduction to the Standard Edition which serves as a justification for his translation of the German '*Trieb*' with the English 'instinct' instead of 'drive'. Most notable, however, is Strachey's acknowledgment that "in some half dozen instances Freud himself uses the German 'Instinkt', always perhaps, in the sense of instinct in animals" (SE I, p. xxv). For example, Strachey notes that Freud writes, in "The Unconscious" (1915b): "If inherited mental formations exist in the human being—something analogous to instinct in animals—these constitute the nucleus of the Ucs" (SE XIV, p. 195).

to an object, for example, a satisfaction or "quantity" that is fundamentally lost. The lost satisfaction, as object, is the clinical fact that leaves the subject with recourse only to 'hallucination', and therefore representation(s), to support and mark the absence of the lost "quantity"—a 'quantity' which Freud terms *das Ding*, or the "Thing".

The opening of the space of psychical reality derives from the rupture of the smooth instinctual functioning that is characteristic of the organism. In the *Project*, Freud confronts the problem of the organism in terms of the relation of "quantity" to "quality", and the question of how the organism renders quality from quantity. I suggest that the category of 'quality' itself originates a concept of the body as the site of a lost quantity and the site of inscription for memory/forgetting and potential meaning.[2]

In part I of the *Project* Freud writes: "All contrivances of a biological nature have limits to their efficiency, beyond which they fail" (p. 306). His reference point, or paradigm, for such a failure is the "pathological" phenomenon of pain. 'Pain', in Freud's explanation, is a 'quality' that represents in the mind the failure of a "biological contrivance" (as limit) and the subsequent effect in the human organism of a surging forth of excess quantity. Freud writes: "Pain is thus characterized as an irruption of excessively large Qs [quantity] into [impermeable neurons] and [permeable neurons]" (p. 307). Pain, then, is a "quality", a representation in the mind, which indicates that a biological contrivance has failed to regulate the organism.

When the organism is not at "degree zero" (homeostasis), it is in "pain". Paradoxically, pain is itself a representational limit that indicates that the biological limit of homeostasis has failed and thus unleashed a certain excess 'quantity' into the organism. However, the cause of the excess quantity—and this is evident in Freud's text—is not simply biological, but instead issues from the point of interface between instinct and social demands. In other words, even in this very early text, Freud does not situate the failure of the organism exclusively in terms of the "failure of the biological contrivance".

---

[2] My claim is consistent with Lacan's (1992) remark on Freud's text in *Seminar VII*: "Freud says that the development of the [psychical] apparatus replaces simple quantity by quantity plus *Bahnung*, that is to say, its 'articulation' [in representation] … [and] … *Bahnung* suggests the creation of a continuous way, a [signifying] chain" (p. 39).

Later in the *Project* Freud introduces the question of a symbolic versus a strictly biochemical exchange:

> At first, the human organism is incapable of bringing about the specific action [to reduce tension]. It takes place by *extraneous help*, when the attention of an experienced person is drawn to the child's state by discharge along the path of internal change. (p. 318)

In the corresponding footnote Freud says that the "discharge along the path of internal change" is manifest "by the child's screaming". Freud continues:

> [T]he discharge acquires a secondary function of the highest importance, that of *communication*, and the initial helplessness of human beings is the *primal source* of all moral motives. (p. 318)

Thus Freud situates the necessary failure of the economy of instinct in the moment of the child's first address to the parental other. However, the scream, as a first instance of the address for help to the parental other, underscores both the initial inarticulateness of the child's appeal to the other, and the ultimate inadequacy of speech and language to maintain the economy of instinct.

Here we can elaborate Freud's observation: the infant *(infans)* is, by definition, 'without speech', yet is subjected to the social imperative to "communicate" his need for satisfaction to the other, e.g., the mother or father. The infant is situated in a linguistic environment where access to physiological satisfaction is mediated by representation, thus subjecting the infant's 'need' to the other's desires(s), whim, and possible refusal. Thus homeostasis is interrupted by requirements imposed by the other: requirements that, given the infant's lack of access to the faculties of reason or understanding, are perceived by the infant as capricious and without sense. The correspondence between the loss of satisfaction and the lack of sense or justification for the loss is fundamental. [3]

---

[3] Lacan offers an important observation on Freud's *Project*, precisely on the question of "pain" as a limit in the mind, a signal, that the "unpleasure" principle has failed. In *Seminar VII* Lacan says that "we should conceive of pain as a field which, in the realm of existence, opens precisely onto that

In the *Project*, we have the primary forces that cause the subject and raise the question of ethics as defined in the Introduction, e.g., the failure of the organism and the human's dependency on speech and language which are inadequate to stand in, or account for, the lost quantity.

2.2.2 Instinkt versus Trieb

Freud's interrogation of the gap between 'instinct and its object' will provide us access to the body of drive. In the *Three Essays* Freud provides an analysis of the nature of instinct and its relation to the object. In his conclusion to section I of the *Three Essays on Sexuality* (1905), Freud suggests that it was through the consideration of the perversions that he discovered the impossibility of situating instinct (that is proper to the animal) in the human being:

> Experience of the cases that are considered abnormal has shown that in them the sexual instinct [*Trieb*] and the sexual object are merely *soldered* together—a fact which we have been in danger of overlooking in consequence of the uniformity of the normal picture, where the object appears to form part and parcel of the instinct. (Italics added, SE VII, p. 148)

Now, if we understand instinct which is proper to the animal to have a specific cause (stimulus), and an object suited to satisfy the need evoked by the stimulus, then it is clear that Freud has discovered something other than instinct in the human being—the object is merely "soldered" to the instinct. In other words, according to Freud, the instinct seems to have lost its object.

---

limit where a living being has no possibility of escape" (p. 60). Human subject formation implies a radical confrontation between the organism and the Law: a confrontation that is *necessary*, that is, there is "no possibility of escape". Ultimately, it is the primary effects of the Law that the human *qua* 'subject' cannot "escape" and that function as the cause of physiological disequilibrium and thus the source of 'psychical reality' and its 'pain'. However, the psychotic, as opposed to the neurotic, bears a different relation to this 'pain'—that is, 'pain' as a product of the Law. I return to the question of "pain" and the psychotic subject's relation to the Law and social demand in Chap. 6, *Ethics*.

> We are thus warned to loosen the bond that exists in our thoughts between instinct and object. … [T]he sexual instinct is in the first instance independent of its object; nor is its origin likely to be due to its object's attraction. (ibid., p. 148)

In this passage, Freud teases apart the stakes of drive from those of instinct. Thus Freud opens the question of the second body of drive as the result of the organism's subjection to a radical loss of the object, and thus a radical loss of any recourse to a real object, versus a representation, that could satisfy the constant 'thrust' of the drive.[4]

To continue, *Instincts and Their Vicissitudes* (1915a) represents Freud's earliest attempt to systematically describe the structure of the drive. According to Freud, the movement of the drive is structured by the interaction between the thrust (*Drang*), the source (*Quelle*), the object (*Objekt*), and the aim (*Ziel*). In the following passage Freud writes of the pressure of the drive in terms of the "demand for work" upon the mind:

> If we now apply ourselves to considering mental life from a *biological* point of view, and 'instinct' appears to us as a concept on the frontier between the mental and the somatic, as the psychical representative of the stimuli originating from within the organism and reaching the mind, as a measure of the demand made upon the mind for work in consequence of its connection with the body. (SE XIV, pp. 121–122)

With the "frontier between the mental and the somatic" we have a peculiar conflation of inside (organism) and outside ("psychical representation") that points to the problem of locating the body that psychoanalysis is concerned with. I am suggesting that psychoanalysis is in search of a body that is in between the organism and representation, a body that is no longer of the organism, however a body that remains without recourse to representation. Eventually, following Lacan, we will locate this body that is stranded in between, and that is literally in pieces, as the body of the letter. The psychotic knows the body of the letter very well.

[4] This is what Lacan (1978) insists upon in his return to Freud, that is, drive, unlike instinct, is unique to the experience of the "speaking being" as subjected to representation (see "Transference and the Drive", *The Seminar of Jacques Lacan: The Four Fundamental Concepts of Psychoanalysis, Book XI*).

For Freud the production of drive is linked to an irrevocable loss of the object—such that there is no natural object of a so-called instinct as found in the animal-without-language, but instead an object of/for the drive that is "merely soldered" to the drive, which, furthermore, problematizes the traditional notion of satisfaction for the human. The rupture of the organism by the loss of the real object and satisfaction introduces a profound disequilibrium into the human.

In *Beyond the Pleasure Principle* (1920), Freud proposes the hypothesis of the death instinct [*Trieb*], as that which is beyond, and contradicts, the pleasure principle as a function of biology, for example, as evidenced, according to Freud, in the phenomenon of the repetition compulsion. In contrast to a repetition compulsion that operates in accord with the pleasure principle, Freud locates instances where the repetition compulsion appears as pure death drive beyond the pleasure principle—a repetition that is outside the logic of instinctual satisfaction.

> [T]he compulsion to repeat also recalls from the past experiences which include no possibility of pleasure, and which can never, even long ago, have brought satisfaction even to instinctual impulses which have since been repressed. (SE XVIII, p. 20)

Death drive represents the failure of the pleasure principle as the biological imperative that regulates, Freud had assumed (up to this point), the physiological organism and "mental life". Freud writes of the necessity to posit the death drive and the repetition compulsion in order to account theoretically for what remains beyond the pleasure principle:

> Enough is left unexplained to justify the hypothesis of a compulsion to repeat—something that seems more primitive, more elementary, more instinctual than the pleasure principle [which it overrides]. (p. 23)

In the face of the clinical fact of the "perpetual recurrence of the same thing" Freud confirms the necessity of the hypothesis of the death drive and the repetition compulsion. Following Freud, and given that the organism and its pleasure principle are "overridden", the subject is left with recourse only to social Ideals and imperatives (Language) to fashion a limit to the death drive unleashed in, and forming, the 'body-in-pieces'.

2.3 The Impact of the Other on the Organism: Drive after Lacan

Lacan's reading of Freud's drive theory discovers the true consequences for the organism of its confrontation with the demands of the social world. For Lacan, the body, as opposed to the organism, is the surface that bears the effects (e.g., erogenous zones, mnemic traces, the 'letter') of Language and speech. In *Seminar XI (1981)*, in his reading of Freud's *Instincts and Their Vicissitudes*, Lacan rescues drive from instinct and shows how the structure of drive is in no way a natural phenomenon, but instead a structure caused in the moment of the organism's subjection to the field of the social Other, e.g., to Language and social "Demand". The point for Lacan, here, is to throw into question the meaning of satisfaction vis-à-vis the structure and terms (thrust/source/object/aim) of the biologically based concept of drive.

Specifically, Lacan interrogates the premise that "the satisfaction of the drive is reaching one's *Ziel*, one's aim" (p. 165). Lacan says that, instead, "[t]he aim is the way taken [by the drive]" (p. 179). In other words, for Lacan the aim is not the attainment of the object of satisfaction as in the case of hunger in the animal, but instead the path the drive takes around the lack of a real object, and therefore the path the drive takes in spite of the impossibility of satisfaction itself.

A central implication of Lacan's intervention is that drive is rendered as a phenomenon that is the effect of social forces on the organism. Drive is no longer understood to indicate, as with the traditional interpretation of Freud's psychosexual stages, the instinctual force behind a biological (maturational) process that culminates in the formation of a body organized and totalized under the 'genital zone'. Lacan says:

> The passage from the oral drive to the anal drive can be produced not by a process of maturation, but by the intervention of something that does not belong to the field of the drive—by the intervention, the overthrow, of the demand of the Other. (p. 180)

With the "intervention of the demand of the Other" Lacan introduces the experience and effect on the body of the threat of castration and the Law:

> The threat of castration is like a thread that perforates all the stages of development. It orientates the relations that are anterior to its actual appearance—weaning, toilet training, etc. It crystallizes each of these moments in a dialectic that has as its center a bad encounter. (p. 64)

The dialectic that structures the so-called developmental stages is the dialectic of subject and Other—what Lacan calls the Symbolic[5] Other. I am suggesting two conceptions, or versions, of the Other that structure the psychical life of the human: the "Other of demand" and the "Other of desire". This distinction bears consequences in (1) regarding the place of the subject in the structure of language and the "address" (subject and Other), and (2) concretely, regarding the psychical experience of the child in the social nexus of family–society (e.g., the subject's subjection to Ideals and cultural requirements). For the child, the Other of demand is represented by the figure of the "Imaginary" (uncastrated/unlimited) father vis-à-vis the mother–child dyad. In contrast, the Other of desire is represented by the symbolic father, as a desiring and thus a lacking and castrated Other.

Lacan, in *Seminar IV, The Object Relation* (1994), locates the Imaginary father as the agent of "privation". "Frustration, privation, and castration" represent three varying relations to the lost object, or 'object a' cause of desire. In the psychic life of the subject, the imposition of a loss (castration) by the imaginary father is experienced as capricious. The passage

[5] The Symbolic order is one of the three registers (with the Imaginary and Real) that Lacan deploys to understand psychic experience. The Symbolic register, or order, includes the cultural requirements (rules of coexistence) and sociocultural demands that impact, and ultimately produce, the subject.

through the fantasy of Imaginary castration differs markedly for the psychotic versus the neurotic. In the course of the formation of the subject of neurosis, the ideals of the family (Oedipus) are articulated to the Ideals of culture. In other words, for the neurotic, the loss incurred at the hand of the Imaginary Other is inscribed in the realm of cultural–symbolic exchange, and is thus supported and legitimated by the desire of the Other. I suggest that it is the Imaginary Other of demand that the psychotic confronts alone, due to a failure of a necessary articulation. The problem of articulation will be addressed in terms of the return and "break-in" of the voice in the experience and phenomenology of psychosis.

I will now situate the distinction between the Other of demand and the Other of desire within the context designated here as the dialectic of 'body and organism', and in terms of the psychotic experience. Clinically, I would say that the 'Other of Demand' introduces the new subject to the violence, and trauma, of language. It is in the very installation of the dialectic of subject and Other (S→O) that the organism sustains the first cut, or loss. The first encounter with the Other that introduces the cut is traumatic precisely because the cut is sustained without justification and without the choice of the individual. In short there is no signifier for the Other's demand; demand simply leaves its mark as a trace of the subject on the body. In terms of psychosis, we can say that the voice in hallucination is an effect of the Other of pure demand. The Other of demand, represented in the psychotic's experience of the voice, is a capricious Other that is by definition without limit. Recall that the psychotic is often commanded by the voice to kill themselves; or else the voice severely ridicules the subject, and, in the context of the delusion, elects the subject to serve an all-powerful Other (e.g., God or a government agency).

In contrast, the 'Other of desire' introduces, into the life of the subject, the function of negation through the necessity of symbolic castration, or limit. The signifier of the Other's desire, and therefore of negation itself, is the "phallus". The phallus, as signifier of the primary loss/lack introduced by demand, functions to support the subject in his or her pursuit of the lost object of desire. Key here, particularly in terms of psychosis, is that the phallus represents the incompleteness of Language and, in the unconscious of the human, represents the limit placed on the power and capriciousness of the Other of demand. I will expand on the importance of the negative function of the phallus later.

To conclude on the question of the body of drive, one could say, following Lacan, that the Freudian drive constitutes a *silent* response to the demand of the Other. Freud says in *Beyond* (1920) that death drive is "silent". This Lacanian point regarding the effect of social demand is not far from the Freudian notion of "instinctual renunciation" as a requirement of "civilization". Lacan is simply returning to a fundamental question raised by Freud, namely, how does a given subject reckon with, and respond to, the cultural requirement of a radical loss of access to satisfaction?

However, we have to extend this question to include the clinical fact that the said requirements of civilization, including cultural ideals, and the Law/limit, carry with them no true justification. The question of justification, or lack thereof, opens the way for further clarification between (1) a conception of language as purely traumatic versus (2) a conception of language (signification) as that which allows the subject to bear the real of the trauma.[6] In neurosis, the subject bears the real, or truth, of the trauma via the mechanism of repression, and through the articulation of the Ideals of the Ego to the Ideals of society. Given the psychotic's *Verwerfung* (foreclosure), what is the psychotic's position vis-à-vis the double function of Language?

In *After Lacan* (2002), psychoanalyst Danielle Bergeron writes of the function of the Law, represented by the symbolic "Father", as a function that establishes the limit between the possible and the impossible. It is important to note that theoretically the limit marked and sustained by the Father function is a universal limit, or Law applicable to all. But, as Bergeron notes, the true status of the paternal Law-as-universal-limit, and therefore the status of symbolic castration, is sustained by a "fiction", that is, the limit is purely symbolic and thus unfounded.

---

[6] The distinction between Language as 'trauma' (versus symbolic barrier) is addressed later in terms of the relation of "justification" (for loss) to the "paternal function". This distinction, and its consequences for the psychotic, is further elaborated in terms of repression versus *Verwerfung* (foreclosure).

> [T]he symbolic Father is also a fiction that in Language sustains a meaning for life by repressing the absence of any justification for loss, that traumatism at the root of the human experience. (p. 72)

So, following Bergeron, the instinctual renunciation as the requirement of symbolic castration is without "justification". This clinical fact is repressed for the neurotic. In other words, for the neurotic the "fiction", the symbolic Father, functions to repress, as Bergeron puts it, the "emptiness of meaning in human existence—a confrontation that would rend one's world apart" (p. 73). In contrast, the subject of psychosis faces the Void, the Absence, an emptiness where meaning would be anchored and sustained. It is only because the body of the human is carved from the organism that he must face the problem of making meaning, and Sense. In particular, the psychotic faces the questions of life and death without the benefit of the barrier of the symbolic function to repress the primary and unjustifiable cost of entering into the rules of language and coexistence. The cost is linked to what Bergeron refers to in the previous quote as the "traumatism at the root of human experience".

Again, on the subject of drive and 'maturation', Lacan says:

> There is no natural metamorphosis of the oral into the anal drive. Whatever appearances may emerge to the contrary from the play of the symbol constituted ... by the supposed anal object, namely, the feces, in relation to *the phallus in its negative effect*, we can in no sense—experience shows us—consider that there is a continuity between the anal phase and the phallic phase, that there is a relation of natural metamorphosis. (italics added, pp. 180–181)

The "phallus in its negative effect" implies castration, a loss. Symbolic castration requires a loss in/of the organ(ism) to the symbol (phallus). But, if we follow Lacan here, the negation, manifest in the appearance of the phallus in the psyche, does not occur in the course of a natural maturational process. Rather, the Symbolic meets the organism with pure violence, as pure trauma. For example, Lacan notes in *Seminar XI* that the unconscious itself is the effect of a pure negation, the effect of an "original

Un, namely, the cut" (p. 43). The said "cut" is none other than the traumatic loss of satisfaction introduced by Language.

> I saw a profound link between this cut and the function as such of the subject, of the subject in its constituent relation to the signifier [language] itself. (p. 43)

The phallus, as a corollary of the Symbolic Law, is installed in the psyche and functions as a barrier, a limit, to the primary violence introduced by the Other of Language and social demand. Key here for Lacan is that the movement of drive towards the phallus—the phallic stage in Freud's terms—is (1) dialectical and (2) at base caused by an encounter with violence and trauma, or a "bad encounter" with Language and the demand of the Other. The body of drive represents a failure of the instinctual functioning of the organism.

- What is the status of the *subject* in relation to the body?

In the context of the present study, the term "subject" implies the 'subject of the unconscious' produced by the effect of language and of repression (e.g., a 'primary' repression or original 'cut'). For example, one is born subject(ed) to the pre-existing desire of parental others, and the demands of one's culture. We have to refer again to Lacan's articulation of the original cut that produces the subject. Lacan says there is a "profound link between the cut and the function as such of the subject" (p. 43). More specifically, it is the very site of impact on being, and on the organism, of the Other's desire (a negation) that constitutes the subject of the unconscious. Hence Lacan's reference to an original "Un" or negation that leaves its mark as the trace of the subject.

On the question of subject formation psychoanalyst Lucie Cantin (2002) notes in "'The Trauma of Language":

> [T]he human subject is a creature of language. For humans, the most natural of events, such as birth and death, are wholly caught up in the symbolic web created by language. […] Long before conception one is born a sub-

> ject, subjected to the discourse and the desire that resulted in one's conception and birth. (p. 37)

The subject is birthed in the moment of the organism's traumatic encounter with Language. The subject is born, in other words, in the moment of the failure of the organism. The failure implies the mapping of drive over instinct and the introduction of an unconscious logic of the body in opposition to the bio-logic of the organism.

Freud's introduction of the failed "contrivance" in the *Project* and his theory of biology's limit in *Beyond* foreground the following questions: Where does the said failure situate the subject, as itself an effect of the failure, in relation to the question of the limit on excess? And, specifically regarding psychosis, how does this failure manifest (i.e., return) in the body of the psychotic, and in the structure of the psychotic experience?

2.4 Apollon, Bergeron, and Cantin: The Return of the Lost Object in the Body of the Psychotic

2.4.1 The Internal Object

It is often said that the problem of the psychotic is that she has *not* lost the object. As Jacques-Alain Miller (2002) writes in "La clinique d'ironie", "[p]sychosis is the clinical structure in which the object is not lost, in which the subject has it at his or her disposition". However, insofar as there is a version of the 'Other' in psychosis, there must also be a fundamental loss through which an Other may come into being. I will show that the difference for the psychotic is that the loss is incurred without representation or symbolic articulation, and thus without justification or exchange value. The object is lost, but not, as in neurosis, to a system of exchange regulated by symbolic rules. It is worth noting again that this supposed lost object is nothing in particular, but instead represents a Thing that the subject and members of a community encounter as lost or lacking.

The effect of the excess that returns in the body of the psychotic can be witnessed in the presence of the "internal object", and the phenomenon of the voice, in the psychotic's elaboration of their experience. Typical examples of the internal object in the phenomenology of psychosis include "electronic devices" installed in the body for the purpose of receiving orders via an auditory hallucination to carry out a mission in the service of an omnipotent Other, e.g., the White House or NASA. Following Lacan, the first object in the psychoanalytic sense is the voice. Thus we might begin by understanding the 'voice', a primary object, as representing the traumatic "break in" of the Other of language into the being, or fullness, of the organism. There is a link, then, between the internal object and the voice that commands the psychotic.

In "Dream and Jouissance" (2002), Daniel Bergeron explains the function of the internal object in terms of the relation of symptom to delusion:

> In psychosis, the symptom appears as the subject's resistance to the Other's demand for jouissance. It situates inside the body a knot of jouissance and partializes this knot within the body. (p. 83)

The symptom in psychosis functions as a solution to an impasse resulting from a contradiction between the imperative of satisfaction and the imperatives set forth in the discourse of delusion. The internal object, Bergeron notes, constitutes the point of resistance to Demand and castration, a "knot of jouissance," i.e. prohibited satisfaction.

> [T]he psychotic's symptom sets itself up as an irreducible, unassimilable rock of jouissance piercing delusion which would proclaim the imaginary existence of an Other who, filled out by the psychotic, does not lack. (p. 84)

The internal object is, as Bergeron phrases it, the "partialized knot within the body". Note the homophonic relation of knot to 'not' as indicative of the negating effect of the internal object vis-à-vis the psychotic delusion. As 'k/not', a point of resistance, the internal object functions to problematize the otherwise smooth functioning of the delusion. For now, we could say that the internal object represents the k/not, an internal contestation, of the delusion and the failure of the symptom to negotiate the contradiction between a satisfaction required by the subject and the demand for jouissance from the Imaginary Other.

Psychoanalyst Willy Apollon (2004),[7] in a lecture entitled "On Psychotic Structure", explains that the status of the "voice", as obscene and omnipotent, in the psychotic's experience/phenomenology is an effect of a failure in subject formation to link the voice—which is the "father's" voice—to a "name and a face". Apollon says that "[the link between] the word, the face, the voice and the name rests upon the good word of the mother". The function of the mother's "good word" is to name the father of and for the child. Apollon underscores the problematic of the first link between the word and the thing—such that for Freud, as opposed to linguists, "the relation between the word and the thing is libidinal". Note that the mother's "word", in 'naming' the father, designates a desirable, and thus libidinally invested, third term. The failure of the linkage between the "good word" of the mother and the installation of the name (of the father) leaves the psychotic without the necessary libidinal-symbolic link, or 'function'. Apollon says: "The Name of the Father [a symbolic function] is the *first example of all human life*, where the name, the voice, the word, and the face are fundamentally linked." We will follow Apollon further on this last point in the following chapter. However, I will explore the question of the relation between the lost/"internal" object and the fundamental libidinal-symbolic link between word and thing (absence and presence) in terms of Freud's discovery in the *Project*, and Lacan's elaboration in *Seminar III*.

Once the status of the psychotic's body is thus linked to the question of the 'choice' of the psychotic regarding castration and loss we find once again the question of fantasy and the first hallucination that supports desire. This, in turn, links the internal object to the question of the radically lost object—the 'object a' as cause of desire/lack, and cause of the subject.

Bergeron's location of the internal object as a point of resistance to Demand and Imaginary castration is fundamental to the notion that the

[7] Apollon, W. (2004, February). *On psychotic structure*. Lecture delivered in the context of the "Clinical Cases Seminar in Puerto Rico". Hosted by the Puerto Rico Psychoanalytic Circle of the Freudian School of Quebec. San Juan, Puerto Rico.

psychotic's body is itself a site of social contestation. The presence of the internal object concerns the status of the relation between the voice, the Other of language, hallucination, and the problem of perception. We must situate the problem of the "internal object" in relation to the question of hallucination—not only the phenomenon of auditory hallucination (e.g., the persecutory voices) typical of the psychotic experience, but also in relation to the fundamental hallucination that intervenes to support the advent of the subject in the encounter with an originating cut, or break-in, of language and the Demand of the Other. In Freud's *Project* we find that the function of a first hallucination, an object of desire, stands in for the lost object of need. The hallucination serves as an 'aesthetic act' by the subject that is designed to substitute for the loss of the "real" object. The capacity to hallucinate, the hallucination itself, masks the pure absence laid bare at the moment the infant discovers the lack opened up by the failure of satisfaction and the economy of need. In the field of psychosis, however, it is not a question of whether or not the psychotic loses the object (the "thing"), but rather of the psychotic's specific relation to what is a *necessary* loss of the thing: for the psychotic, the question regards why the loss is 'unbearable'.

2.4.2 Hallucination in the Production of the 'internal object'

As discussed earlier, in the *Project* Freud approaches the function of hallucination as a mechanism required to fill the gap left by the failure of the "experience of satisfaction". Freud locates the human being as stranded in between a failed biology and the inability of language to satisfy need. "The human organism is incapable of bringing about the specific action [to reduce tension]" (318). And, as noted, the "child's scream" or cry is but a first, and inarticulate, attempt to alert the parental other to the effect on the child of the parental other's absence (i.e., as cut). However, the child's cry merely evokes, renders audible, the child's fundamental relation to the lack of satisfaction, and frustration, born from the encounter of need with the original negation introduced by Other of language.

The task of the infant-subject, in the moment of a possible subjective collapse provoked by the absence, is to produce a fantasy, or more accurately a hallucination, to take the place of the absence of the parental other and the subsequent frustration of need. Freud is clear when he states that the place of veridical perception, for the speaking being, is replaced by wishful fantasy or hallucination.

> Thus, as a result of the experience of satisfaction, a facilitation comes about between two mnemic images and the nuclear neurons which are cathected in the state of urgency. (p. 319)

The "experience of satisfaction" is, by Freud's own definition, supplemented by the wish, the hallucination, and thus constitutes an experience of failure and lack. The "mnemic image" is but a trace or a mark in the psyche that evokes the impossibility of satisfaction. The "experience [or hallucination] of satisfaction" is something that is installed, and thus "reproduced", as Freud says, in the face of the demand characteristic of the "state of urgency"—in other words, in response to the constant thrust of the drive. The drive, unlimited or unbarred, produces a state of urgency.

> [T]he mnemic image of the object will be the first to be affected by the *wishful activation.* I do not doubt that in the first instance this wishful activation will produce the same thing as a perception—namely a *hallucination.* (p. 319)

Freud's "mnemic image of the object" is a precursor to his later formulation of a "perceptual identity" that sustains subsequent 'experience(s) of satisfaction'. In Chapter VII of *The Interpretation of the Dreams (*1900), Freud writes of the problematic nature of satisfaction vis-à-vis the "continuous" internal pressure of the "somatic"—of the drive.

> [T]he situation [somatic needs] remains unaltered, for the excitation arising from an internal need is not due to a force producing a momentary impact but to one which is a continuous operation. A change can only come about if in some way or other (in the case of a baby, through outside help) an 'experience of satisfaction' can be achieved which puts an end to

> the internal stimulus. An essential component of this experience of satisfaction is a particular perception … the mnemic image of which remains associated thenceforward with the memory trace of the excitation produced by the need. As a result of the link that has thus been established, next time this need arises a psychical impulse will at once emerge which will seek to re-cathect the mnemic image of the perception and to re-evoke the perception itself, that is to say, *to re-establish the situation of the original satisfaction.* (italics added, pp. 565–566)

A link is established between the mnemic image and the memory, not the "perception itself", of satisfaction. The "essential component" of the experience of satisfaction (a "particular perception") is in fact, according to Freud's logic, non-existent—there exists only a memory of the perception of satisfaction. Freud continues and describes how the "wish" functions to support the recurrence of the experience of satisfaction:

> An impulse of this kind we call a wish; the reappearance of the perception is the fulfillment of the wish; and the shortest path to the fulfillment of the wish is a path leading direct from the excitation produced by the need to a complete cathexis of the perception. (pp. 565–566)

It should be clear that, for Freud, there is a difference between the "re-evocation of the perception of satisfaction", the "perception of satisfaction", and "satisfaction itself". If we follow Freud on this point, it would seem that the "wish" and "hallucination" function to repress, *to make bearable*, the absence of the perception of "satisfaction itself". Freud concludes the following:

> Nothing prevents us from assuming that there was a primitive state of the psychical apparatus in which this path [from excitation to perception] was actually traversed, that is, in which wishing ended in hallucinating. Thus the aim of this first psychical activity was to produce a 'perceptual identity'—a repetition of the perception which was linked with the satisfaction of the need. (p. 566)

Freud posits a linkage, and thus a gap, between the perception re-evoked by the wish and subsequent hallucination, and the possibility, in a "primitive state", of a direct path from excitation to perception, i.e., satisfaction.

The psychotic bears a particular relation towards satisfaction and its absence. Satisfaction, following Lacan, is on the side of jouissance and thus always represents a total satisfaction, which, by definition, is prohibited and impossible for the speaking being. The appearance of hallucination in the "first psychical activity" marks the installation of the barrier, for the human, between the possible and the impossible. As the primary psychical, and thus aesthetic, act of the subject, hallucination is linked to what Lacan terms a 'first signification' that marks the lack opened by the failure of satisfaction itself.

2.4.3 Object A: The voice

What relation does the psychotic have to the problem of a first hallucination-signification that, we assume, functions as a support for the subject? Again this keeps open the question of the psychotic's relation to a primary loss. As discussed earlier, in psychosis the fundamental loss of the object is, in fact, incurred—however, the loss is incurred without representation and thus without justification or exchange value. An understanding of the status of the psychotic's relation to the lost object of the drive (the 'object a' in Lacan's terms), and it's relation to the "internal object", hinges upon an elaboration of this last question regarding loss and its "representative".

2.4.4 Internal Object, Object A, and Representation: Writing on the Body

In *The Language of Psychoanalysis* (1973), Laplanche and Pontalis, reading Freud, attempt to understand (1) how the body of drive finds its "representative", and (2) the specific "nature" of the representative as a "delegate of the instinct" (pp. 203–205). The authors also note that the establishment of the first representative of the "instinct" is contingent upon the linkage of "primal repression" and "fixation"—a fixation, it would seem, of the representative to the "instinct" that has been denied access to consciousness. In "Repression" (1915c), Freud describes the linkage between the dual functioning of primal repression and fixation:

> We have reason to assume that there is a *primal repression*, a first phase of repression, which consists in the psychical (ideational) representative of the instinct [*Trieb*] being denied access into the conscious. With this a *fixation* is established; the representative in question persists unaltered from then onwards and the instinct remains attached to it. (SE XIV, p. 148)

Freud theorizes the ideational representative, not simply as a content of the unconscious, but as constitutive of the unconscious as topological space. The relation of primal repression to fixation functions as the process by which the unconscious itself is constituted.

As Laplanche et al. note, Freud links the notion of fixation with inscription—the inscription of the "instinct" [*Trieb*] in the unconscious—as the mode by which the perception is registered. In *Letter 52* of the correspondence with Fliess, Freud terms the inscription of perception as the "indication of perception"—the 'indication' constitutes a "first registration" (i.e., *Niederschriften or* "writing down") of the event of primal repression (SE I, pp. 233–239). The primary inscription functions as the 'object a', and a "writing down" of the loss or cut that constitutes the unconscious as such.

2.4.5 Psychotic 'Inscription': The Purely Traumatic versus the Nominative Function of the Word

The fact of 'inscription', which constitutes the object a, is key; but the location of the precise function of inscription itself is essential if we wish to answer the question of the psychotic's relation to the lost object. Laplanche and Pontalis underscore the difficulty of locating the status of the inscription when they raise the question of the "nature of the ideational representative". Let us, by contrast, say that the "nature" of the representative is to mark, or delimit, the unconscious and its "instinct" as that which is radically lost, and thus impossible. This makes the body, as

I am defining it, an effect of this inscription or letter. The body is of the letter/inscription, which in turn leaves the question of the representative of the loss, or inscription, to one side.

The category of "unconscious" or "instinct" is best considered empty of content regarding the event of primal repression, and what Freud terms the "first registration". The unconscious here is situated on the side of what Lacan terms the original "Un" or negation that establishes the category of the prohibited, and therefore the constitution of an inaccessible zone. The first registration, or inscription, is the mark of a purely formal injunction introduced by the Other of language that splits being, and thus creates the primary condition for the advent of the "divided" subject. So, when Freud writes that "[primal repression] consists in the psychical (ideational) representative of the instinct being denied access", we are confronted with, as Freud says, a moment or event that functions as the cause of the subject that must be "assumed" to have occurred, although it is an event that may only be deduced after the fact.

In *Seminar III, The Psychoses* (1993), Lacan comments on how Freud considered the institution of the Symbolic and the Law:

> If Freud insisted on the Oedipus Complex to the extent of constructing a sociology of totems and taboos, it is obviously because for him the Law is there *ab origine*. It is therefore out of the question to ask oneself the question of origins—the Law is precisely there from the beginning, it has always been there, and human sexuality must realize itself through it and by means of it. This fundamental law is simply the law of symbolization. (p. 83)

For the human, Language as trauma simply exists—the trauma of Language is there "ab origine". However, I posit that the necessity of Language (a pure Demand/imperative), as constitutive of the human condition, does not presuppose the Law (the "order") of symbolization. In the "Function and Field of Speech and Language", Lacan (1977) isolates the specific relation of the Law to the ordering of society:

> This law, then, is revealed clearly enough as identical with an order of language. For without kinship nominations, no power is capable of instituting

> the order of preferences and taboos that bind and weave the yarn of lineage through succeeding generations. (*Ecrits*, 1977, p. 66)

Thus there is no "order of language" without the Law, without "nomination" [the name/first signifier], the function of which is to designate the possibility of order itself. The nominative, versus traumatic, function of Language common to neurosis occurs *après coup* or 'after the blow' that is common to the advent of every subject. The psychotic's discourse is evidence of the non-existence of the Law, i.e., the order, or the nominative function, of the signifier is not functioning in psychosis. For the psychotic there is no articulation of loss to the logic of the Symbolic Law, and thus she/he confronts psychoanalysis with the problem of 'origins' and of justification. The psychotic's delusion, her entire enterprise, is constructed around the question of origins and the ultimate lack of a satisfactory response from the Other/other to such a question.

Freud and Lacan both suggest that the assumption or supposition of the event of primal repression and its symbolization are required to begin an inquiry into the experience and structure of subject formation in psychosis, neurosis, or otherwise. With the psychotic subject, however, Lacan shows us that we confront the question of a radical failure of repression and symbolization, i.e., symbolization of an event that we can only suppose to have happened.

Lacan frames the problem of the origin or advent of the neurotic versus the psychotic subject, and structure, in terms of the difference between, and implications of, two psychical mechanisms: *Verdrangung* (repression) and *Verwerfung* (foreclosure). As I noted in the Introduction, Lacan theorized that the psychotic structure is determined by a radical exclusion ("foreclosure") of the primary word, or "signifier", that, for neurotic subjects, provides a first link in the subject's effort to make sense of experience. This leaves the psychotic without the primary, or fundamental, symbolic link to anchor the structuring of psychical reality. The mechanism of foreclosure destabilizes the epistemological foundation for the limits, rules, and social contracts that structure symbolic and consensual reality.

However, here we are concerned with a fact, a necessary event, that lies behind the mechanism of foreclosure. The problem for the psychotic subject in its relation to psychical and symbolic reality regards what Lacan, following Freud, terms a "primordial *Bejahung* (affirmation)". In *Seminar III* Lacan says: "In the beginning, there is either *Bejahung*, which is the affirmation of what is, or there is *Verwerfung*" (p. 82). This leaves the mechanism of repression to one side for the moment. Foreclosure, then, constitutes a refusal of a necessary affirmation of what is, of what may exist specifically in the Symbolic.

Lacan says:

> Prior to all symbolization—this priority is not temporal but logical—there is, as the psychoses demonstrate, a stage at which it is possible for a portion of symbolization not to take place. (p. 81)

For Lacan the logical problem concerns the advent of the subject and its coincidence with the event of the institution of the symbolic Law, and its effect. But with the psychotic, we deduce that the subject has refused, from the symbolic chain, the credible foundation for the Law (i.e., its "representative") thus excluding a symbolic barrier to jouissance.

> This initial stage precedes the entire neurotic dialectic, which is due to the fact that neurosis is articulated speech, insofar as the repressed and the return of the repressed are one and the same thing. It can thus happen that something primordial regarding the subject's being does not enter into symbolization and is not repressed, but rejected. (p. 81)

Fundamental to Lacan's observation is the designation of the status of the Symbolic Law, and thus the subject itself, as either "articulated in speech" or not. The "neurotic dialectic", as Lacan phrases it, presumes the subject's confrontation with the stakes of Oedipus and castration. For the neurotic the trauma of language is repressed, inscribed in the Symbolic, and thus rendered meaningful. In neurosis, the primary loss (of jouissance) in the encounter with the Other's Demand is dramatized (made meaningful), we could say, in the fantasy that structures the 'Oedipus complex'. The point, here, is that the object that structures the fantasy of Oedipus is an object that has been irrevocably lost. However, in the field of neurosis, Oedipus 'articulates' (justifies), retroactively, the fundamentally unjustifiable status of the loss.

The work of analysis attempts to articulate the logic of the subject's solution to an otherwise meaningless and, as noted earlier, "unjustifiable" loss introduced by language. Thus what is inscribed, and subsequently repressed (for the neurotic) by the Name-of-the-Father, is a non-sensical 'sign' or 'letter' (not a signifier) indicative of the event, or cut, of language. The psychotic, by contrast, faces the Void opened up by the primary cut without a first signifier to mark and support the absence of the Thing. The psychotic is stranded without the "libidinal" link between word and thing that could render the Void between word and thing unknown (repressed) and thus bearable.

2.5 Conclusion: One Psychotic Object

We must assume, then, that the subject of psychosis lives according to another logic—in other words, according to a logic that operates without recourse to the affirmation of existence that serves as the fundament, the base, for the symbolic life of the neurotic subject. This brings us back to the specific question of the internal object. Lacan's formulation "that something primordial regarding the subject's being does not enter into symbolization ... but [is] rejected" is instructive. For now we can link the status of the internal object to the "rejection" of that which might symbolize and justify the lost quantity of 'being' required/demanded by the Other. In its various manifestations, the internal object represents the status of the Demand of the Other as without limit, or reach, regarding the subject. Thus, the voice as object is experienced by the psychotic as internal—as an internal object that speaks, against which the subject has no defence except to submit to and serve the Demand of the voice.

References

Apollon, W. (2004, February). *On psychotic structure. Lecture delivered in the context of the "Clinical Cases Seminar in Puerto Rico." Hosted by the Puerto Rico Psychoanalytic Circle of the Freudian School of Quebec.* San Juan, Puerto Rico.

Bergeron, D. (2002). The work of the dream and jouissance in the treatment of the psychotic. In R. Hughes & K. R. Malone (Eds.), *After Lacan: Clinical practice and the subject of the unconscious* (pp. 71–85). SUNY Press.

Cantin, L. (2002). The trauma of language. In R. Hughes & K. R. Malone (Eds.), *After Lacan: Clinical practice and the subject of the unconscious* (pp. 35–47). SUNY Press.

Freud, S. (1895). *Project for a scientific psychology*. In J. Strachey (Ed. and Trans.), *The standard edition of the complete psychological works od Sigmund Freud* (Vol. I). Hogarth Press, 1999: 283–397.

Freud, S. (1900). *The interpretation of dreams.* SE Vols. IV&V, 1999.

Freud, S. (1905). *Three essays on sexuality*. SE Vol. VII, 1999: 135–243.

Freud, S. (1915a). Instincts and their vicissitudes. SE Vol. XIV, 1999: pp. 114–140.

Freud, S. (1915b). "The unconscious." SE XII, 1999: pp. 159–216.

Freud, S. (1915c). Repression. SE Vol. XII, 1999: pp. 141–158.

Freud, S. (1920). *Beyond the pleasure principle.* SE XVIII: 1999, pp. 3–63.

Lacan, J. (1977). The function and field of speech in psychoanalysis. *In Ecrits: a selection* (A. Sheridan, Trans.). W.W. Norton & Co.

Lacan, J. (1978). *The four fundamental concepts of psychoanalysis, the seminar of Jacques Lacan, Book XI* (J.A. Miller, Ed., and A. Sheridan, Trans.). W.W. Norton & Co.

Lacan, J. (1992). *The ethics of psychoanalysis (1959–1960), The seminar of Jacques Lacan, Book VII* (J.A. Miller, Ed., and D. Porter, Trans.). W.W. Norton & Co.

Lacan, J. (1993). *The psychoses (1955–1956), The seminar of Jacques Lacan, Book III* (J.A. Miller, Ed., and R. Grigg, Trans.). W.W. Norton & Co.

Lacan, J. (1994). *La relation d'objet.* Text established by J.A. Miller. Seuil.

Laplanche, J., & Pontalis, J. B. (1973). *The language of psychoanalysis.* W.W. Norton & Co..

Miller. J.A. (2002). A Contribution of the Schizophrenic to the Psychoanalytic Clinic (La clinique d'ironie). E. Ragland & A. Pulis (Tr. & Eds.). Retrieved September 25, 2005, from http://www.Lacan.com/newspaper2.htm.

3

The Impasse of Transference in Psychosis

3.1 A Question Preliminary to the Provocation of Transference

The central concern of this chapter is the problematic of the "installation" of the transference in the field of psychosis. A primary objective of installing the transference is to establish a new *opposition* in the psychic life of the psychotic.[1] Both Freud and Lacan found that psychoanalysis (a practice which rests upon the successful provocation of transference) ran aground on psychosis. It is important to locate precisely where, and why, Freud and Lacan determined that transference reached an impasse with the psychotic. What Freud and Lacan found, I argue, is that the psychotic will not enter the transference via the neurotic mechanism of identification with the analyst as the one supposed to know. The demand for love that characterizes the neurotic's position in analysis is radically absent from the psychotic's demand, and thus the subject supposed to know is

[1] The function of the dream vis-à-vis the installation of transference is the topic of the next chapter. However, here, I provide a brief note on the nature of the "opposition". The 'opposition' is in fact between different knowledges—different structures (e.g., the structure that is lacking (dream) versus a structure without lack (delusion). The dream is opposed to delusion insofar as the dream functions according to the laws of language whereas delusion does not.

B. Fimiani, *Psychosis and Extreme States*, The Palgrave Lacan Series,
https://doi.org/10.1007/978-3-030-75440-2_3

not presumed by the psychotic to be on the side of the analyst. The absence of the demand for love is a consequence of the primary psychical mechanism operative in psychosis: *Verwerfung* (foreclosure). What does the psychotic's *Verwerfung* of the fundamental "libidinal tie" (the Name-of-the-Father) imply regarding the impasse of transference? I argue that the impasse of transference hinges upon the question of the psychotic's *Verwerfung* and its consequences.

Thus the primary task of this chapter is to follow Freud and Lacan on this last point. The impasse Freud and Lacan reach with the psychotic is instructive insofar as the impasse functions as a guide to understanding the shift required in the position of the analyst to provoke and sustain the transference with the psychotic.

3.2 Freud: The Psychotic Subject as Itself an Obstacle to Transference (*Classically Defined*)

Why does Freud conclude that the psychotic had "no capacity for transference" (SE XVI, p. 447)? In *Lecture XXVII* (1917a) entitled "Transference," Freud provides what perhaps is his clearest account of the problem the psychotic presents for psychoanalysis. Departing from a description of the efficacy of psychoanalysis in the treatment of the neuroses Freud writes:

> There are, however, other forms of illness in which, in spite of the conditions being the same, our therapeutic procedure is never successful. These patients, paranoiacs, melancholics, sufferers from dementia praecox, remain on the whole unaffected and proof against psychoanalytic therapy. (SE XVI, pp. 438–439)

It is interesting that Freud locates both "melancholics" and "sufferers from dementia-praecox (schizophrenics)" as hopeless subjects of psychoanalysis—the psychotic as "proof" against the psychoanalytic cure. Freud designates melancholics and schizophrenics as hopeless precisely because, as he says, they are "incapable of a libidinal object cathexis" (p. 446). In both melancholia and psychosis we have a specific mode of failure to re-cathect or find a substitute for some(thing) radically lost. Thus Freud observes that the problem for the psychotic vis-à-vis transference regards the subject's particular relation to the loss of the object. The "libidinal object" is the lost object, or Lacan's 'object a'. I have already begun to establish that the psychotic has a specific relation to the lost object. I have argued that the psychotic's "internal object", a particular manifestation of the libidinal lost object, indicates a short-circuiting of the Symbolic Other's place in the psychic life of the psychotic (see Chap. 2).

There is a consequence of this manoeuvre by the psychotic. For the psychotic, the Other is not installed as the one who is perceived and positioned by the subject to possess the lost object. In contrast, with the neurotic for whom the object is lost to symbolic exchange, the neurotic's position implies not only that an Other has "justifiably" acquired the object, but also, and this is key regarding the neurotic transference, that it is an Other who is *supposed to know* something about the loss that carves out the lack/desire that causes the subject itself. *It is a question of the place/location of the object for the subject.* The psychotic, according to Lacan, has no question, she *knows*. In other words, the psychotic is certain about the place of the object and the function of the Other. The psychotic does not question or doubt the place of the object or, more importantly, the status of the Other's desire vis-à-vis the lack of an object.

Freud's discovery, with the melancholic and schizophrenic, prefigures the Lacanian formulation of the psychotic's relation to the lost object and the Other's desire/lack. In *Lecture XXVII* (1917a) Freud refers to the psychoses and melancholia as "narcissistic neuroses". As Laplanche and Pontalis (1973) note, the key point here is that the term 'narcissistic neurosis' implies both an "impossibility of libidinal transference" and a "withdrawal of libido onto the ego" (p. 258). Freud (1917a) writes:

> Observation shows that sufferers from the narcissistic neuroses have no capacity for transference or only insufficient residues of it. They reject the doctor, not with hostility but with *indifference*. For that reason they cannot be influenced by him either; what he says leaves them cold, makes no impression on them; consequently the mechanism of cure which we carry through with other people—the revival of the pathogenic conflict and the

> overcoming of the resistance due to repression—cannot be operated with them. They remain as they are. (italics added, SE XVI, p. 447)

Freud's designation of the psychotic's "indifference" will function as our guide in the effort to find what is at stake for the psychotic in the installation of the transference.

Freud locates the failure of transference in the "indifference" of the psychotic to the doctor (analyst)—the analyst "leaves them cold, makes no impression on them". Of particular import is the distinction Freud observes between "hostility" and "indifference". In the previous quote Freud locates the psychotic on the side of indifference, thus excluding the psychotic from the opposition that constitutes the hazard common to the neurotic transference. For example, regarding neurosis, Freud sees the affective (including the "erotic" and the "negative") transference as both a potential obstacle and what is essential to the analytic cure of the neuroses: "Transference can arise as a passionate demand for love; in place of a wish for love" (p. 442). In "Observations on Transference-Love" (1915) Freud writes the following regarding the handling of the "erotic" transference in neurosis:

> To urge the patient to suppress, renounce or sublimate her instincts the moment she has admitted her erotic transference would be, not an analytic way of handling them, but a senseless one. It would be just as though after summoning up a spirit from the underworld by cunning spells, one were to send him down again without asking him a single question. (SE XII, p. 164)

The appearance of the "erotic" versus the "negative/hostile" transference corresponds to the neurotic's perception of a confirmation or refusal of the object suited to satisfy the "demand for love". The central point here regards the function in neurosis of the demand for love itself. In neurosis the patient's demand positions the analyst as the one with the power (i.e., the knowledge) to refuse or grant the neurotic's wish (demand) to be loved/hated, and thus completed.

What Freud finds in the encounter with the psychotic is, by contrast, the absence of a demand for love: the psychotic's "indifference". Thus,

Freud argues, "The mechanism of the cure … cannot be operated with them" (p. 447). Freud finds that the analyst has no leverage; the mechanism of transference-love fails to function with the psychotic. Without the "pathogenic [i.e., Oedipal] conflict" or "resistance due to repression", the transference misfires. Freud misses the encounter with the psychotic subject by confronting psychosis with a model of transference structured fundamentally by the encounter with the neurotic. If the stakes of transference are simply Oedipal the psychotic is left stranded in a field of indifference to the other (the analyst). The psychotic, in contrast to the neurotic, does not position the analyst as the one supposed to have, or to know, what the analysand should want or be. For now let us simply say that the so-called indifference represents a radical lack of desire and, most importantly, the analyst's failure to provoke desire (or a question, a lack) on the side of the psychotic. A failure, then, of transference.

For the missing solution to the problem of transference in psychosis, Freud substituted a sustained desire to know the configuration, and thus the true stakes, of the psychotic experience. Freud's impasse with the psychotic is instructive insofar as the impasse itself underscores Freud's recognition of psychosis as an experience radically different in its structure from neurosis—an experience that psychoanalysis had yet to successfully enter (clinically).[2] "They remain as they are", as Freud says. Freud's modesty will lead us towards a solution for the impasse of transference with the psychotic. Freud discovers that the psychotic's own solution by way of delusion presents new difficulties for psychoanalysis and, in particular, the mechanism of the transference. Freud points us towards a solution for the transference impasse in the psychotic patient when he ends the passage in *Lecture XXVII* (1917a) regarding the indifference of the psychotic with the following:

> Often they [sufferers from narcissistic neuroses] have already undertaken attempts at recovery on their own account which have led to pathological results. We cannot alter this in any way. (p. 447)

[2] Except via Freud's theoretical analysis in the case of Daniel Paul Schreber (1911).

What 'cannot be altered' by the classical neurotic analytic position, Freud recognizes, is the "attempt at recovery", its very form—in the "symptom". Freud's use of the term symptom is equal to what I have termed the phenomenology of psychosis. For example, the psychotic's fundamental experience is represented in the phenomenology, i.e., the functioning of the voices and the delusion structure a unique relation of the subject to the trauma. Here Freud has discovered, in part, the importance of the psychotic's delusion as "symptom".

In *Notes on a Case of Paranoia* (1911) Freud writes:

> The delusional formation, which we take to be the pathological product, is in reality an attempt at recovery, a process of reconstruction. (SE XII, p. 71)

What is the precise difference that lends the psychotic's "symptom" its distinction? The difference, and Freud was clearly aware of this, is that the symptom in psychosis (i.e., the delusion) regards a unique knowledge about the agent of castration and its consequence—the lack of an object of satisfaction. This has a significant consequence for understanding the position of the analyst in the transference, and fundamentally what the psychotic's *Verwerfung* ("foreclosure") implies. Foreclosure, defined as the exclusion of a fundamental libidinal investment, is, as Freud puts it in his reading of the *Schreber Case*, an "internal catastophe", and the end of a "subjective world" (p. 70).

> The patient has withdrawn from the people in his environment and from the external world generally the libidinal cathexis which he has hitherto directed into them. … The end of the world is a projection of an internal catastrophe; his subjective world has come to an end since his withdrawal of his love from it. (p. 70)

The "internal catastrophe" again calls forth the nature of the psychotic's primary, and originary, encounter with Language. The "internal catastrophe" is an effect, or result, of a radical exclusion/refusal, versus the repression, of a primary "representative". For the psychotic there is a failure of primary repression and symbolization to shield the subject from the traumatic inscription of the Other's Demand.

3.2.1 The Failure of a Fundamental Libidinal Tie and Its Consequence for Transference

It is generally understood that the psychotic, or subject of psychosis, inhabits her psychical structure in a particular way that is distinct from that of the neurotic or the pervert. The psychotic strikes a different position in relation to the said trauma of Language and to castration. Following Lacan, I suggest that the position of psychosis (a psychical structure) is the result of a 'choice' vis-à-vis the problem introduced by the trauma of language, the disruption of the organism, and the subsequent eruption of death drive that, in turn, composes the fragmented body. This initial choice is the "forced choice" that is made for the speaking being in its confrontation with Language. So, to begin, we could say that the initial choice that defines the psychotic's position is the choice that is inherent in the mechanism of foreclosure. What is foreclosed for the psychotic is the installation of symbolic castration itself.

Situating the structure of psychosis as the result of a fundamental choice makes sense only within the context of the clinic. Why? It is only within the context of clinical treatment, under transference, that the psychotic can then establish the conditions necessary to contest the pathological effects of their initial choice vis-à-vis the trauma. *I will show that, ultimately, the "installation" of transference introduces the question of desire and thus castration into the field of psychosis.* It is desire-as-barrier-to-jouissance that is "installed" by provoking the transference, defined as a 'desire to know', on the side of the psychotic. The opening of the transference presents the psychotic with a second choice regarding their position as subject versus their position as object of the jouissance of the Other-in-delusion. The problem, for the psychotic, is that of creating a path through transference towards a new position for a subject. The question then becomes 'what are the necessary conditions to gain access to the subject of the unconscious of the psychotic?'. This last question is the link between my conception of the body of the psychotic and the problem of the installation of the transference in the treatment of psychosis.

Of course, one might argue, that this is only our reading of Freud *after* Lacan. However, as I have shown in Chap. 2, Freud clearly distinguishes between the "first registration" of the event of primal repression and the libidinal investment in a "representative" of the trauma or 'cut' that is constitutive of the unconscious and of the 'body' itself. The point, if we read Freud closely, is that the psychotic's "internal catastrophe" betrays a knowledge of the catastrophe, or lack of sense, internal to language and the rules that define cultural requirements: to turn Freud's term, the psychotic suffers from an *internal[ized]* catastrophe. The "internal catastrophe" results from the failure to invest libidinally in what Freud terms the "representative" of the "first registration". Thus the psychotic does not repress, through the investment in a "representative", the non-sense or void circumscribed by the Law. The psychotic bears, at the subjective level, some Thing that can only be dealt with collectively. In other words, the psychotic bears the responsibility of the structural failure of language without recourse to a first (master) term or "representative". Where the neurotic enters a love relation through the libidinal investment in the "representative", the psychotic remains alone without the libidinal investment to sustain Oedipus as an explanatory device. The psychotic's position, alone in the face of the void, requires the delusion, as opposed to the Oedipal fantasy, to explain what is not "fixed" to primary repression, and to explain what they know about the lack in language. The psychotic's specific knowledge (*savoir*) requires that the analyst occupy a different position vis-à-vis the "internal catastrophe" and the attempt at "reconstruction" and "recovery" of the object via delusion.

In *Lecture XXVI* (1917), "The Libido Theory and Narcissism", Freud writes of the function of the psychotic's "symptom" and the relation of the symptom to the libidinal object:

> The clinical picture of dementia praecox ... is not determined exclusively by the symptoms arising from the forcing away of the libido from the objects and its accumulation in the ego as narcissistic libido. A large part, rather, is played by other phenomena, *which are derived from efforts of the libido to attain objects once more and which thus correspond to an attempt at restitution and recovery.* (SE XVI, italics added, p. 422)

Freud begins with the premise that the phenomenology of psychosis is determined by the effort via delusion to "attain objects once more". We must assume that the effort by the psychotic differs from that of the neurotic. Of course, all symptoms, whether neurotic or psychotic, aim to attain the object of satisfaction. In "On Narcissism" (1914) Freud, by contrast, writes of the specific nature of the neurotic's libidinal tie:

> A patient suffering from … neurosis has also, as far as his illness extends, given up his relation to reality. But analysis shows that he has by no means broken off his erotic relations to people and things. He still retains them in fantasy; i.e., he has, on the one hand, substituted for real objects imaginary ones from his memory, or mixed the latter with the former; and on the other hand, he has renounced the initiation of motor activities for the attainment of his aims in connection with those objects. (p. 74)

Freud articulates the precise difference between the withdrawal of libido in neurosis versus psychosis. The "paraphrenic" (paranoiac or schizophrenic) is characterized by "megalomania" and "the diversion of their interests from the external world—from people and things" (SE XIV, p.74). "Megalomania", the total withdrawal of libido onto the ego and from symbolic exchange, renders the psychotic, as Freud says again here, "inaccessible to the efforts of psychoanalysis" (p. 74).

It is clear that, for Freud, the status of the transference hinges upon a given subject's relation to the other vis-à-vis the lost libidinal object. The nature of the libidinal tie to the other depends upon the status of the lost object for the subject.

> It is otherwise for the paraphrenic. He seems really to have withdrawn from people and things in the external world, without replacing them with others in fantasy. When he *does* so replace them, the process seems to be a secondary one and to be part of an attempt at recovery, designed to lead the libido back to objects. (author's italics, p. 74)

With the term "secondary" Freud implies the secondary (versus primary) process and, by extension, the function of the "word presentation" versus the "thing presentation" respectively. Freud's frequently cited observation, that in psychosis the word <u>is</u> the thing, applies here. In other words, Freud's formula (word <u>is</u> thing) speaks to the collapse of the gap between word and thing that separates representation from the object or 'thing' represented. This last point situates the problem of transference in psychosis as one of a lack of a 'lacking object'—and thus a lack of desire in the psychoanalytic sense. *The effect of the collapse between word and thing, paradoxically, does away with the thing as such.* If we take Freud literally when he says that in psychosis the word *is* the thing, then there is no category of the impossible. The status of the lost object in neurosis, in contrast, suggests such a category or limit.

If we return to the passage from *Lecture XXVII* we can begin to understand the stakes for the psychotic in the face of transference.

> It seems as though in dementia praecox the libido, in its efforts once more to reach objects (that is, the presentation of objects) does in fact snatch hold of something of them, but, as it were, only their shadows—I mean the word presentations belonging to them. (p. 422)

The psychotic structure is determined by the failure of a first libidinal link between the word and the thing. Of course the link itself implies a gap instituted by the primary repression of this fact, i.e., the fact that the link between the word and the thing is merely libidinal is precisely what is repressed in neurosis. For the neurotic the loss is symbolized and stabilized through the repression of the non-sense that links the word to the thing. Recall that by "the link between the word and the thing" we mean the replacement via representation of the thing with the word. As Lacan puts it, "the word is the murder of the thing", thus rendering the thing as that which is radically lost. But this formula, or knowledge, is the product of the "neurotic dialectic" in which there is, in fantasy, a lost thing or quantity for which the word is a mere representation or, as Freud puts it, a mere "shadow". The position Freud assumes here, again, confronts the psychotic with a neurotic epistemological framework.

Most important for our understanding of transference is that the dialectic of desire and love is not installed in psychosis. We only have to recall a simplified version of Lacan's formula that, fundamentally, desire is the Other's desire in order to see the problem for the psychotic. Desire is desire for the thing that is lost. And yet, finally, we are not saying, either, that the psychotic has not lost the object, but only that the psychotic bears a different relation to the lost object—the object as 'lack' in the Other, which translates, for the psychotic, as the Other's Demand for jouissance. This question has been illustrated earlier in terms of the status of the object as "internal".

3.3 Lacan and the Impasse of Transference in Psychosis

I want to return to the main thesis of this chapter which suggests that the installation of transference is equal to the installation of symbolic castration or, more accurately, equal to the installation of the *effects* of symbolic castration as such. This has particular relevance in the treatment of psychosis given that, as I have argued earlier, the psychotic does not necessarily pass through the dual neurotic mechanism of identification, or love. This is the problem with treating the psychotic as Freud saw it. In place of an identification with, and libidinal investment in, the analyst, through which the neurotic may repeat the structure of a fundamental libidinal tie/investment, Freud observed that the psychotic meets the analyst with a certain "indifference".

3.3.1 The "Transference Effect" Versus the "Subject Supposed to Know"

Towards the end of *Seminar XI* Lacan (1978) articulates the stakes of transference in terms of the dialectic of the "[subject] supposed to know" and the "desire of the analyst". "As soon as the subject who is supposed to know exists somewhere … there is transference" (p. 232). In this text, Lacan is aiming at understanding the stakes for the neurotic, not the psychotic. However, as with Freud, by way of Lacan's theory of the neurotic transference we can better understand the stakes for the psychotic. It must be noted that although Lacan remains in the field of neurosis, he takes us further in our attempt to establish a theory and practice of transference that provides access to the 'subject of the unconscious' versus a model of transference that strands the patient in an identificatory relation to the analyst.

Lacan is careful to warn against any conception of the analytic cure (transference) as founded on a 'dual' relation: "Love [a narcissistic/dual relation], no doubt, is a transference effect, but it is on its resistance side" (p. 253). Transference, for Lacan as well as for Freud, requires the dialectic composed of (1) "love" (as narcissistic investment) and (2) that which lies 'behind' the "transference effect": the 'desire to know'. Lacan says:

> [W]hat is there, behind the love known as transference, is the affirmation of the link between the desire of the analyst and the desire of the patient. (p. 254)

The point, though, is that transference, as demand for love, is the entry point for the neurotic patient into the analytic experience. The neurotic patient's demand for love will collide with the desire (lack) of the analyst.

Thus, in the field of neurosis,

> [w]e are linked together awaiting this transference effect in order to be able to interpret, and at the same time, we know that it closes the subject off from the effect of our interpretation. (p. 253)

The "link" between "the desire of the patient and the desire of the analyst", however, is supposed by the analyst and is based only upon the existence of the demand for love. In other words, the demand for love itself betrays the desire (the radical lack of satisfaction) that the fantasy of a dual (complete) relation is designed to obscure. This is what Lacan means by 'supposing the subject' (of desire), i.e., with the neurotic, behind the demand for love we suppose a desiring subject with a singular knowledge.

Lacan's insistence upon the subject provides a reference point regarding the question of transference in psychosis. As Lacan says, "[t]he transference is unthinkable unless one sets out from the subject who is supposed to know" (p. 253). The "subject" supposed to know *is* the subject of the trauma, but what does this imply? Thinking through the problematic of neurosis, Lacan poses a key question: what, exactly, is the "subject" supposed to know? In other words, *what does the subject itself know*? In *Seminar XI* Lacan suggests the following answer:

> He [the subject] is supposed to know that from which no one can escape, as soon as he formulates it—quite simply, signification. Signification implies, of course—and that is why I first brought out the dimension of his desire—*that he cannot refuse it*. (italics added, p. 253)

So Lacan argues that we must begin with the subject of the unconscious: a subject that is defined by a knowledge of radical subjection to the signifier. This raises the question of a distinction, key to this discussion, between 'subjection' (pure trauma) and 'castration' (in the symbolic register). The register of the said "subjection" is important. I want to be clear that it is not the subject that is subjected insofar as the subject itself is the effect of subjection to a Demand implied by Language. As I have argued in Chap. 1, the subject is the effect of the subjection of the *organism* to the signifier—the subject is constituted by a pure knowledge of the death introduced by the signifier, or word.

However, in the following passage, Lacan introduces the necessity of an "absolute point with no knowledge". Again we see the requirement of the "neurotic dialectic" in order for transference to function.

> This privileged point is the only one by which we can recognize the character of an absolute point with no knowledge. It is absolute precisely by virtue of being in no way knowledge, but the point of attachment that links his very desire to the resolution of that which is to be revealed. (p. 253)

This last quote immediately follows the phrase "that he [the subject] cannot refuse it". The "privileged point", the "absolute point with no knowledge", functions as an "attachment". I suggest that the "point of no knowledge" designates the functioning of the neurotic mechanism of repression, which thus implies the installation of the Name-of-the-Father. The Name-of-the-Father, as signifier and justification of the Law, is the "privileged point" in the Symbolic *par excellence*. The Name-of-the-Father is also a signifier about which the subject of neurosis remains necessarily ignorant, such that in order to maintain repression the status of the Name-of-the-Father, itself non-sensical, must remain unknown.

Lacan continues:

> The subject comes into play on the basis of this fundamental support—the subject is supposed to know, simply by virtue of being a subject of desire. (p. 253)

The subject appears, "comes into play", on the basis of an ignorance essential to neurosis, for example, the subject, and thus the unconscious, emerges in the dream, parapraxis, and so on, all of which constitute unconscious productions that by definition require the mechanism of repression.[3] Unconscious productions are addressed to the Other that, as Lacan argues, the subject "cannot refuse".

But isn't it the mechanism of foreclosure that implies that the subject may in fact "refuse it [a first signification]"? The subject of psychosis is constituted by the knowledge inherent in the experience of "refusal" (*Verwerfung*) of the first signifier—thus the psychotic is alone in a universe where the possibility of a symbolic limit on the Other's Demand has been 'refused'. This last point requires a distinction that is implied but not fully articulated in the text of Lacan.

1. Both the subject of neurosis and psychosis are the effect of a subjection of the organism to the signifier. But the question of the subject's submission to symbolic castration is subsequent, I suggest, to the trauma—hence opening the possibility of repression versus foreclosure.
2. Only the subject of psychosis 'chooses' to refuse the Name-of-the-Father as guarantor, thus forgoing repression and complicating the question of desire for the psychotic.

[3] This last point raises a question concerning the precise difference regarding the function of the dream in neurosis versus psychosis. If we accept that the provocation of transference hinges upon the appearance of the dream, then what is the status of the "dream-work" for the psychotic given the primacy of foreclosure (of the Ideal) over repression? This question will be addressed in the following chapter.

Insofar as desire implies symbolic castration, the question of whether or not the psychotic is a "subject of desire" prior to transference, defined as a desire to know, remains an open question. Lacan locates the problem of foreclosure as the primary obstacle to installing a desire to know *in* psychosis. In the remaining sections of this chapter I focus on the relation between 'foreclosure' (of a libidinal tie represented in the Name-of-the-Father) and its consequences in the effort to establish transference.

3.3.2 Psychosis: The Limit of Transference

Similar to Freud, Lacan makes several definitive statements that indicate his hesitation in the face of psychosis and the possibility of its treatment. But, as I indicated earlier, it is important to understand the logic of Lacan's position here. "On a Question Preliminary to Any Possible Treatment of Psychosis (1977)", which chronologically follows Lacan's extensive study of psychosis in *Seminar III* (1993), is devoted to keeping the question of the *treatment* of psychosis, in the most radical sense, open. The "question" that is preliminary, Lacan tells us, is the question of the "defect [foreclosure] that gives psychosis its essential condition". Lacan makes the following remark at the end of the "On a Question Preliminary …":

> To say that on this terrain [psychosis] we can do anything would be premature, because it would now be to go 'beyond Freud' … At least that is what separates me from any other object than to restore access to the experience that Freud discovered. (Ecrits, p. 221)

Lacan's final remark in this text is:

> For to use the technique that he [Freud] established outside the experience in which it was applied, is as stupid as to toil at the oars when the ship is on sand. (Ibid., p. 221)

Lacan warns against applying psychoanalysis "outside the field to which it was applied". And, it should be made clear, the "field" to which Lacan refers earlier *is* neurosis. It is certain that Lacan advanced the understanding of the structure and true stakes of the psychotic experience, e.g., in

Seminar III. However, on the question of treatment, Lacan did not reach far beyond Freud's conclusion, particularly regarding the problem of transference. It is true, as the previous quote implies, the analyst cannot reach the "outside" that *is* psychosis if the analyst remains reliant upon "technique", as Lacan puts it, derived from an encounter within the field of neurosis. This last point will be explored in Chaps. 5 and 6, less in terms of "technique" than in terms of ethics.

What does the field of psychosis present to psychoanalysis that, for Lacan, rendered any attempt at treatment "premature" and, in addition, indicative of going 'beyond Freud'? In light of Lacan's positing of the treatment of psychosis as "beyond Freud", I would add the following question: Does the treatment of psychosis require a mutation of psychoanalysis itself—perhaps a reorganization of the fundamental precepts of psychoanalysis in order to properly receive the discourse of the psychotic? The psychotic confronts psychoanalysis with a specific knowledge (*savoir*) regarding Language, its castrating effect, which is fundamentally different from the knowledge offered by the neurotic. Thus I am asking: what is the effect of the psychotic's *savoir* on the structure of psychoanalysis? If we follow Lacan, following Freud, on this last question, it is evident that at this point in Lacan's thinking psychosis represents something radically outside the practice of psychoanalysis. The structural relation of psychoanalysis to psychosis, regarding the question of treatment, is one of exclusion.

In "On a Question Preliminary …" Lacan provides a clue to the primary obstacle that stands between the psychotic and the emergence of a true analytic cure:

> Following Freud I teach that the Other is the locus of that memory he discovered and called the unconscious, a memory that he regards as the object of a question that has remained open in that it conditions the indestructibility of certain desires. (*Ecrits*, p. 215)

Lacan outlines, in part, the fundamental experience that psychoanalysis confronts in the field of neurosis. The "indestructibility of certain desires" implies desire itself, a fundamental lack that in turn functions as the cause of the subject. Note that this is an encounter, a 'supposed' event, i.e., in neurosis, repressed by the Name-of-the-Father. Memory requires repression and, I suggest, therefore that the memory Lacan refers to earlier is not just any memory but the memory as representative of the advent of the subject.

The question of a "memory" vis-à-vis a fundamental lack/desire is key. In neurosis, the "Un", the negation that causes the unconscious, receives, Lacan says, a proper Name which articulates the lost object that constitutes the subject as lacking within Language and symbolic exchange. Without the Name, however, the Other (the Other of Language and the unconscious) that Lacan invokes cannot be the locus of "that memory that he [Freud] discovered and called the unconscious". The limit, marked by the Name-of-the-Father that constitutes the forgetting (the memory) is the Law itself. The Name-of-the-Father, as Lacan says, is "the signifier *in* the Other" and "the signifier *of* the Other as locus of the Law" (Ecrits, p. 221). For the psychotic, the horror of the trauma that for the neurotic is repressed and thus forgotten (a "memory") is perpetually present and manifest, for example, in the abusive and controlling voices characteristic of psychotic phenomena.

The theoretical context of these quotes is of great importance. In essence Lacan is establishing the precondition for the subject of psychoanalysis and for transference. Lacan argues that psychoanalysis, if we follow the teaching of Freud, requires that "the Other is the locus of that memory … [that is] … the object of a question". The memory of the trauma is the 'object of a question', thus the subject is a subject by way of having a question—in other words, by lacking knowledge about loss. It is important to maintain a distinction here between 'loss' (the trauma itself) and symbolic castration, which, by contrast, implies repression and signification.

3.3.3 The Implication of the Mechanism of "Foreclosure"

It is well known that Lacan locates the "foreclosure" of the Name-of-the-Father as the defining psychical-symbolic event that functions as the cause of psychosis. The Name-of-the-Father indicates the existence of a fundamental, or first, signifier that functions to symbolically found what Lacan terms the "paternal [i.e., Oedipal] function", which, as discussed in Chap. 2, is a symbolic function that legitimates a loss of being in the human. Ultimately the operation of foreclosure introduces a lack into the paternal function. What is lacking in the paternal function due to foreclosure is the link that articulates parental lack to cultural exigencies.

Given its relevance to resolving the problem of transference in psychosis, I must reiterate a key distinction articulated in Chap. 2, with the following question in mind: What is the relation between the Name-of-the-Father and repression? On the topic of the psychotic's relation to the lost object, I argued that the operation of foreclosure leaves the psychotic without recourse to a first signifier to protect the subject from the capriciousness of the Other's Demand. I suggested that it is in the work of psychoanalysis that the analysand attempts to articulate the logic of the subject's solution to an otherwise meaningless and "unjustifiable" loss introduced by language. Thus what is inscribed, and subsequently repressed for the neurotic by the Name-of-the-Father, is a non-sensical sign or letter (not a signifier) indicative of the event, or cut, of language. However, the psychotic, given the primacy of foreclosure, faces the Void opened up by the primary cut without a first signifier to mark and support the absence of the thing (or total satisfaction). The psychotic is stranded without the "libidinal" link between word and thing that could render the Void between word and thing unknown (i.e., repressed) and thus bearable. So, the Name-of-the-Father is synonymous with the operation of repression—the repression of the trauma and the lack of Sense introduced by the trauma.

The important point, regarding the link between the Name-of-the-Father and repression, is that primary repression creates an 'inaccessible zone' about which the individual, versus the subject, can know nothing. It is in fact the inaccessible knowledge regarding the object of the trauma that is subsequently supposed to the Other and, specifically, to the person of the analyst. For Lacan, like Freud, the possibility of transference, and thus treatment, requires that the patient misrecognize the analyst as the one who knows. More accurately, the analyst is supposed by the neurotic patient to have access to knowledge that the patient does not. The misrecognition of the analyst supposes that the patient is under the sway of

Oedipus—insofar as Oedipus provides a figure, an image, and a narrative, to explain the lack of Sense that is itself traumatic. Oedipus supposes a trauma, the knowledge of which is imputed to the analyst. This operation is constitutive of the love relation that is basic to the neurotic transference. "If you [the analyst] love me, you will protect me from what I do not know about that (trauma/truth) which causes me as subject". I suggest that, for Lacan, this fundamental split, caused by primary repression, functions as a prerequisite for transference. The Name-of-the-Father is implied because the Name-of-the-Father functions as a guarantee and, most importantly, lends a sense to the trauma of a non-sensical loss.

In strictly Lacanian terms, then, the provocation of transference depends upon the successful installation of the Name-of-the-Father and thus the successful repression of the ultimate meaninglessness of castration, i.e., in the absence of the repression guaranteed by the Name-of-the-Father, the operation of castration is laid bare as pure trauma, as pure violence. With the failure of symbolic castration we witness, recalling Freud's term, the end of the psychotic's "subjective world" due to an "internal [or internalized] catastrophe". The central point, as observed earlier with Freud, is that, for the psychotic, there is no question of an appeal to the Other (or analyst) for a symbolic barrier to protect the subject from the effects of the catastrophe—a catastrophe, I have argued, that is inherent to Language and its demand for work. If foreclosure implies the exclusion of the very possibility of a symbolic limit, and thus the impossibility of a symbolic place for the object, then what could the analyst offer the psychotic as an alternative to the psychotic's own solution, via delusion, to the catastrophe?

3.3.4 The Non-existence of Symbolic Castration and the Psychotic's Knowledge of this Experience

In "On a Preliminary Question ..." Lacan designates the possibility of treatment, via the installation of transference, wholly contingent upon the mechanism of foreclosure:

> … I will leave this question [of foreclosure] that is preliminary to any possible treatment of the psychoses—a question that introduces, as we see, the conception to be formed of the handling, in this treatment, of the transference. (Ecrits, p. 221)

Lacan insists that foreclosure, and its consequences, require further inquiry and understanding prior to any formalization of a psychoanalytic approach to treatment. I would suggest that Lacan's juxtaposition of the problem of foreclosure (the relevance and fundamental importance of this 'defect'), with the installation of desire in psychosis, constitutes the main axis, or dialectic, that for Lacan maintains the impasse regarding the problem of transference in psychosis. This last observation is consistent with the logic of our discovery reading Freud on the same question. The analyses of Freud and Lacan suggest that the impasse in transference with the psychotic hinges upon the failure of a primary libidinal tie with a "representative". The question for the purpose of the present argument becomes: "what is the relevance of the fact of foreclosure of the Name-of-the-Father to the question of transference?" And, what consequences does foreclosure introduce regarding the position of the analyst and status of the "analyst's desire" as that which provokes the transference (a desire to know) in psychosis?

Lacan argues that with the operation of "foreclosure", the subject refuses representation to that which ultimately cannot be represented. In Chap. 2, I wrote that foreclosure constitutes a refusal of a necessary affirmation (*Bejahung*) of what is, of what may exist specifically *in* the Symbolic. *Bejahung* is the affirmation of what may exist in the Symbolic. *Verwerfung* constitutes the exclusion of what may exist from the Symbolic. With the distinction between *Bejahung* and *Verwerfung* we approach the stakes for the psychotic facing the possibility of transference. But what does the possibility of transference imply given the distinction between *Bejahung* and *Verwerfung*?

I suggest that there are two aspects that figure in the phenomena of existence versus non-existence of what may 'be' in the symbolic. The first is the existence of symbolic castration itself, and the second, which is implied by the first, is the question of the quantity of being excluded by Language and thus rendered non-existent. The non-existent quantity of being is permitted an existence, a place (although in fact it only ex-sists) by way of the installation of the Law. The question then regards the place of being (as lost object) vis-à-vis the Symbolic and thus, I would suggest, the status of symbolic castration.

In *Seminar III* Lacan suggests a relation between *Verwerfung* and castration:

> It can happen that a subject refuses access to his symbolic world something that he has nevertheless experienced, which in this case is nothing other than castration. The subject's entire subsequent development shows that he wants to know nothing about it, Freud literally says, *in the sense of the repressed.* (author's italics, p. 12)

As Lacan observes, for the psychotic there is an "experience". However, one may ask, is the experience one of symbolic castration? The "experience" to which Lacan refers to in this passage, I suggest, is an index of the trauma that every subject encounters—a universal experience. The reference to an "experience" raises the question of the link (a gap) between symbolic castration and the traumatic "experience" itself. The footnote to the previous quote in *Seminar III* leads the reader to Freud's distinction between "rejection" (*Verwerfung*) and repression, and ultimately to the distinction between the existence and non-existence of castration. Freud (1918) writes the following:

> When I speak of having rejected it, the first meaning of the phrase is that he would have nothing to do with it, in the sense of having repressed it. This really involved no judgement upon the question of its existence, but it was the same as if it [castration] did not exist. (SE XVII, p. 84)

What is implied by the non-existence of castration, and what bearing does the non-existence of castration have upon the question of the place of 'knowledge' in psychosis? For both Freud and Lacan repression implies the existence of "castration", and thus, most importantly, the existence of the lost object (representing a lost jouissance/satisfaction). *Verwerfung* (rejection) implies the non-existence of symbolic castration and thus the non-existence of an object (jouissance) that is radically lost. Insofar as the loss/lack, under *Verwerfung*, is not inscribed in the symbolic Other, repression is not functioning. Contrary to its 'exchange function' in neurosis, in psychosis the lost object is not one of exchange, but is instead lodged in the body of the psychotic. She/he *knows* where the object is and why the object is there.

In psychosis, the "experience" of subjection to Language is not repressed through the operation of the signifier of the Name-of-the-Father. Thus we must separate the traumatic "experience" of Language from the repression of the "experience", i.e., it is not clear that we can speak of the existence of castration without the guarantee of repression through the Name-of-the-Father. If castration implies a limit, an operation that renders the "experience" bearable, then it follows that it is premature to suggest that the psychotic knows anything about castration. *Because it does not exist, the supposition of knowledge of castration to the psychotic may only occupy the status of a 'hypothesis' (a question) on the side of the analyst.*

In a later section of *Seminar III* Lacan further clarifies the distinction between *Verwerfung* and repression:

> On the subject of *Verwerfung*, Freud says that *the subject did not want to know anything about castration, even in the sense of repression.* As a matter of fact, in the sense of repression one still knows something about the very thing that one doesn't want, in some sense, to know anything about, the whole of analysis consists in showing us that one [the neurotic] knows it very well indeed. If there are things the patient wants to know nothing about, even in the sense of the repressed, another mechanism is implied. (author's italics, p. 149)

In order to emphasize the psychotic's positive (non-repressed) knowledge of the traumatic "experience" we might rephrase Lacan's statement in the following way: '*the psychotic in fact knows the "experience" itself, and castration (as dependent upon a symbolic mechanism) simply doesn't exist*'. The existence versus the non-existence of castration is not debated in the discourse of the psychotic. The psychotic's delusion, if nothing else, demonstrates a totalizing (uncastrated) knowledge. Castration is not a question in psychosis, as it is, say in perversion where the mechanism of 'disavowal' only confirms the existence of castration. Deploying Lacan's distinction between opposing knowledges, I contend that prior to transference in psychosis there is no 'desire to know' or, conversely, desire 'not to know'.

This last point brings forth the central difficulty regarding transference and, furthermore, underscores the central thesis being argued in this chapter. I began with the premise that the installation of transference defined as a desire to know depends upon the introduction of castration (i.e., desire itself) into the field of psychosis. However, as the previous analysis indicates, following Freud and Lacan, castration requires the operation of repression and its representative. To be more precise, perhaps we can say that the neurotic cannot face castration except with the mechanism of repression. As psychoanalyst Daniel Bergeron (2002) writes, the paternal function and the Name-of-the-Father "guarantee the limits of jouissance" and sustain the "fiction of meaningfulness on which the neurotic's life rests" ("Dream and Jouissance," p. 73).

However, as stated earlier, we are interested specifically in the installation of the "effects" of castration. The term "effects" implies (strictly) the placement/installment of a symbolic limit on the Other's Demand for jouissance. Note also that we are operating with the premise that neurosis and psychosis constitute two radically different psychical structures. This implies that the aim of treatment is never to replace foreclosure with repression, i.e., repression is contingent upon the operation of the Ideals of the ego. The question of ethics hinges upon this last point. Might there be a distinction, then, between the "effects" of symbolic castration as such and the Ideals that the neurotic must maintain in order to accept the effects? The Name-of-the-Father and the Ideals that justify the loss of satisfaction are not credible for the psychotic. Thus, the final question is: How, by what method, can the psychotic accept the limits imposed by symbolic castration without the "fiction of meaningfulness?" The shift, for the psychotic, towards becoming a subject of speech and desire requires a different "ethic", an ethic without recourse to an Ideal or the "Good" to repress the primary arbitrariness and violence of the interdiction imposed by the Other of Language.

3.4 Conclusion: Two Consequences of Foreclosure

There are two main consequences of foreclosure, and of the non-existence of castration in the psychotic's universe. First, given the failure of a first libidinal tie (with the "representative/NOF"), the symbolic Other is not engaged in the "neurotic dialectic" (Lacan), or "love relation" (Freud). Thus the Oedipal stakes cannot be manipulated by the psychoanalyst to trigger the opening of the transference on the affective plane. Second, as a consequence of the first, the analyst is left with the question of how to engage the psychotic's 'indifference'. How will the analyst manoeuvre if the patient does not suppose the analyst to know? What conditions are necessary for the analyst to assume an ethical position in the confrontation with the subject of psychosis?

References

Bergeron, D. (2002). The work of the dream and jouissance in the treatment of the psychotic. In R. Hughes & K. R. Malone (Eds.), *After Lacan: Clinical practice and the subject of the unconscious* (pp. 71–85). SUNY Press.

Freud, S. (1911). Psycho-Analytic notes on an autobiographical account of a case of paranoia (dementia paranoides). SE Vol. XII, 1999, pp. 3–84.

Freud, S. (1914). On narcissism: an introduction. SE Vol XIV, 1999, pp. 67–104.

Freud, S. (1915). Observations on transference-love. SE Vol. XII, 1999, pp. 97–108.

Freud, S. (1917a). The libido theory and narcissism. SE XVI, pp. 412–430.

Freud, S. (1917b). Transference. SE Vol. XVI, 1999, pp. 431–447.

Freud, S. (1918). *From the history of an infantile neurosis.* SE Vol. XVII, 1999: pp. 3–124.

Lacan, J. (1977). On a question preliminary to any possible treatment of psychosis. In *Ecrits: a selection* (A. Sheridan, Trans.). W.W. Norton & Co.

Lacan, J. (1978). *The four fundamental concepts of psychoanalysis, the seminar of Jacques Lacan, Book XI* (J. A. Miller & T. A. Sheridan, Eds.). W.W. Norton & Co.

Lacan, J. (1993). *The psychoses (1955–1956), The seminar of Jacques Lacan, Book III* (J. A. Miller & Tr. R. Grigg, Eds.). W.W. Norton & Co.

Laplanche, & Pontalis, J. B. (1973). *The language of psychoanalysis.* W.W. Norton & Co.

4

Dream-work Versus Delusion

4.1 The Effects and Consequences of the Dream for the Psychotic

The dream and its function in provoking transference in psychosis is the topic of the present chapter. The following questions will guide the inquiry: What is the structural difference between the dream and delusion? How does the dream function differently in treating psychosis versus neurosis? How does the dream function to open a space for the analyst to act and for the subject 'behind the phenomenology' of psychosis to respond? Finally, why would the psychotic choose the dream over delusion, and what are the stakes of the choice of the dream for the psychotic?[1]

To answer these questions we will rely upon Freud's discovery regarding the function of the dream in *The Interpretation of Dreams* (1900), and the work of GIFRIC[2] in the psychoanalytic treatment of psychosis in

[1] This last question, regarding the 'choice' of the dream (desire) over delusion, will lead us to Chap. 5, the topic of which is the problematic of the ethic of the psychotic (as analysand and subject of desire).

[2] On the question of the dream and its function in provoking transference, I will be referring to the ongoing work of psychoanalysts Willy Apollon, Danielle Bergeron, and Lucie Cantin, all founders

B. Fimiani, *Psychosis and Extreme States*, The Palgrave Lacan Series,
https://doi.org/10.1007/978-3-030-75440-2_4

Quebec City. However, Freud's theory of the dream, similar to his theory of transference, is based upon an encounter with the neurotic's psychical structure. In *The Interpretation of Dreams*, Freud defines the "Unconscious" (versus the "Preconscious") as radically "inadmissible" to consciousness, such that there exists an inaccessible zone, a category of the 'impossible' delimited by repression and its "representative". For us, Freud's discovery raises a critical question, and a potential impasse, given that we have theorized that, for the psychotic, there exists no category of the impossible. This potential impasse, regarding the dream, though, returns us to our thesis, which states that the dream, in psychosis, introduces desire itself, and that, therefore, the choice of the dream presents a specific challenge, and risk, to the psychotic.

Furthermore, following psychoanalysts Apollon, Bergeron, and Cantin, we must begin with the premise that delusion has a specific function, and that, to begin the treatment, the analyst must take what the psychotic says (her delusion) literally insofar as delusion functions as a theory of a 'truth' that the psychotic knows. It is the dream that functions to pierce a hole in delusion, thus creating the possibility for the psychotic to reverse her/his position and question the certainty of delusion. However, the said 'possibility' for a new position for the subject, I suggest, hinges upon the production of an ethic in the face of the 'rupture' introduced by the dream; this last point opens the way to a full exploration of 'ethics' in the following chapters. Finally, it is the said 'reversal' of the psychotic's position, vis-à-vis delusional certainty, that marks the 'installation' of transference defined as a desire to know.

My approach to dream-work in the treatment of psychosis differs from that of Apollon et al. in the following way: whereas Apollon et al., I contend, do not adequately theorize the logical relation of dream-work to delusion, my approach offers a detailed theorization of the underlying 'logic' that renders the language of the dream radically different from the language of delusion. My theorization of the relation of dream to delusion is crucial to understanding the conceptual underpinnings of the approach. Furthermore, I have found no published work by Apollon

---

of GIFRIC and the "The Psychoanalytic Treatment Center for Young Adult Psychotics" (the "388") in Quebec City.

et al. or other analysts that theorizes the clinical implication of ethics via the knowledge inherent to the structure of psychosis itself.

Now, if, as I suggest, the dream introduces desire (lack) itself into the field of psychosis, then what sustains the psychotic in the face of desire, and thus symbolic castration, given the absence of the Name-of-the-Father from the psychotic's universe? In other words, what sustains the Law given that the truth of the Law (its unfoundedness) is not repressed by the Name-of-the-Father and thus maintained by the Ideals of the Ego? Moreover, from what position may the analyst act: what will guide the analyst in a 'field' that is, in fact, Other to the Law?

Willy Apollon provides a starting point to address this last question with his formulation of the analyst's position in terms of the "law of the letter and writing", i.e., the 'letter' ('object a') constitutes a field that is 'Other to the Law'. Danielle Bergeron's conception of the analyst's desire and "maneuver" in the place of the 'object a' is instructive, and will guide our effort to determine the true stakes for the psychotic vis-à-vis her encounter with the analyst's desire and the work of the dream. In contrast to the neurotic, the psychotic bears a different relation to the 'object a' (as primary loss) and thus the stakes for the psychotic in relation to the analyst's desire, and to the dream, are fundamentally different.

4.2 The Dream Introduces a Lack of Satisfaction Into the Psychotic's Experience

4.2.1 Freud: The Impossibility of any Ultimate Satisfaction or "Fulfillment"

In *The Interpretation of Dreams* (1900) Freud conceptualized the "psyche" as composed of three interrelated "systems": the Unconscious, Preconscious, and Conscious systems. Psychoanalyst Lucie Cantin (2002) is careful to observe that the Unconscious, for Freud, is the "driving force … the mnemic trace which strives to structure itself and causes the formation of the dream" (p. 88). Freud writes that "when we consider the dream-wish, we shall find that the motive force for producing dreams is supplied by the *Ucs.*" (p. 541). Although not completely clear in Freud's text, we must maintain a distinction between the 'wish' and the "motive force" itself, as this distinction will prove to be what distinguishes the stakes of the dream for the psychotic versus the neurotic.

As Freud says, the dream (every dream) is traceable to an infantile wish for satisfaction, and, we can now extrapolate, this wish is born of a fundamental loss which itself constitutes the unconscious proper. By 'unconscious proper' I imply the existence of repression and thus some "thing" that is, as Freud terms it, "inadmissible to consciousness". As I discuss in Chap. 3, *in neurosis* the primary negation of Being by Language constitutes the [Un]conscious as such, the "Un", which in turn functions as both the cause ("motive force") of the dream and as the lost object of the wish. More precisely, for the neurotic the primary negation, the "Un", is rendered "indestructible" by its "representative" (the Name-of-the-Father). So, as with the impasse of transference, a question emerges regarding the status of the "motive force" (the "Un") for the psychotic and the consequences of the dream given the status of the "representative" of the "Un" (the trauma) as "foreclosed". Thus we can begin with the following premise: the dream (as opposed to delusion) fails to provide any ultimate satisfaction because its cause, its "motive force", is "indestructible" and, as such, cannot be satisfied via the wish. However, in the case of psychosis, this premise must be modified to account for the foreclosure of the "representative" and, by extension, the consequences regarding the status of the "motive force" in psychosis. In psychosis, the subject travels much further on the "path of wish fulfillment", and thus further towards the "destruction" (satisfaction) of the "motive force".

4.2.2 The Object of Dream Versus the Object of Delusion

If it is repression and its guarantee (representative) that render the Unconscious, as Freud puts it, "indestructible", then the psychotic faces a specific consequence that bears upon her choice of dream versus delusion. Freud (1900) writes the following:

> Thus there are two kinds of unconscious, which have not yet been distinguished by psychologists. Both of them are unconscious in the sense used by psychology; but in our sense one of them, which we term the *Ucs.*, is also inadmissible to consciousness, while we term the other *Pcs.*, because its excitations—after observing certain rules [condensation and displacement], it is true, and perhaps only after passing a fresh censorship, though nonetheless without regard to the Ucs.,—are able to reach consciousness. (SE Vol. V, p. 615)

The lost object, Lacan's 'object a', is the effect of the [Un]conscious that is "inadmissible" to consciousness; thus the neurotic may gain access to her 'wish' (for the object of satisfaction) only through representations and thus in a compromised form. For the neurotic the "Un", or more accurately its repression, is represented and explained (theorized and justified) by Oedipus. Oedipus represents and enforces the cultural necessity of loss itself. Yet Oedipus, its manifestation in the family, ultimately reaches its own limit in its confrontation with society, that is, the real mother and father do not possess absolute control, as their authority is limited by that of society and the rules that structure social coexistence. Therefore, via the fantasy of Oedipus ultimate satisfaction is rendered perhaps desirable yet impossible. The prohibition of Oedipus, or more aptly the stability of the prohibition, sustains a libidinal economy of lack in the neurotic, thus the dream merely (re-)evokes the object of the drive. As Apollon (1991) writes of the neurotic's relation to the lost object and to jouissance:

> In neurosis, the fantasy is linked to a jouissance that is hidden [repressed] in the subject which must be brought to face the law in the analysand's speech. (p. 137)

There is something, a repressed satisfaction, in the neurotic that she 'does not want to know' which, as I argued earlier, paradoxically betrays a certain knowing, and a coming to terms with loss, that we cannot impute to the psychotic.

The status of the "Un", a first negation by Language, differs for the psychotic. In Chap. 2 I argued that, for the psychotic, the 'object' is indeed lost but that it returns as an "internal object" in the body, for example in the form of the obscene and commanding voice. In psychosis, then, the presence of the Real internal object reveals the possibility of a total satisfaction (or access to jouissance) in the psychotic's experience.

Furthermore, we can witness the psychotic's satisfaction in the structure and function of delusion, insofar as delusion functions as a totalizing knowledge and provides the psychotic subject with a fixed place/role that in turn bypasses the question of desire: "what does the Other want?" The psychotic does not enter into the dialectic of love (seduction) where, by definition, the subject, but also the Other/other, is fundamentally lacking. Consequently, it is not only, or even primarily, the psychotic subject who is satisfied by the choice of delusion, but the Other—the Other's Demand for jouissance. The psychotic, via delusion, sets out to repair and satisfy the Other's defect and Demand once and for all. Thus, for the psychotic, the status, and the truth, of the Unconscious as "inadmissible" (as primary lack), is destroyed and ultimately satisfied via delusion. With the psychotic, the dream will not merely (re-)evoke the loss and castration, but will, I contend, introduce desire itself by ultimately, as Apollon terms it, "externalizing" the object, thus creating what Bergeron calls a "proper" object: I suppose a "proper" object to imply an object that constitutes lack as the cause of desire, and an object proper to the unconscious.

4.2.3 The 'Structure' of the Dream Demonstrates the Failure of a Wish

If the dream, for the neurotic, is the "fulfillment of a wish" as Freud clearly demonstrates, then how does the dream, by the same token, ultimately introduce a lack of satisfaction? And, more importantly, how does the psychotic face this lack of satisfaction differently? Arriving at an answer to this question depends upon further elaboration of the symbolic status of the "motive force" of the dream and its relation to what Freud terms the "navel" of the dream; both mechanisms, navel and motive force, correspond to some "thing" inaccessible that is impossible to represent. Freud (1900) writes:

> There is at least one spot in every dream at which it is unplumbable—a *navel*, as it were, that is its point of contact with the unknown. (italics added, p. 111)

The resonance between Freud's phrase ("there is at least one…") and Lacan's formulae of sexuation is instructive. Here, in Freud, we have a principle for the 'dream's castration', or a castration that is 'of' the dream, insofar as the dream (representation) runs aground on the 'cause', the "navel", or the Real. The delusion, by contrast, never reaches such a limit.

We can see an example of the 'dream's castration' in the following clinical example.[3] Prior to the beginning of dream-work under transference, a patient may speak only of messages from their voices and distressing beliefs (aka delusion). At a certain point in the treatment the patient elaborated a first dream only to reach an "unplumbable spot" in the dream-work, a navel, where the patient's 'position' in his own speech is 'undecidable' and thus his subjective position vis-à-vis his 'real father' is revealed to be ambiguous as well. So, there was, in his first dream, an 'unknowable'. The point here is that, given that the dream is structured by an 'unknowable', and thus constitutes a 'desiring structure', the space for the subject (as castrated) emerges. Note that the patient, in the face of the 'undecidable' aspect of the dream, and for the first time in the treatment, expressed doubt; he said, regarding an element of the dream: "I'm not sure if I grab the [steering] wheel or just wake him [father] up".

With the dream, then, we have a method of wish fulfilment that must fail given its 'cause'. The dream's 'cause', we might say, 'returns', in the form of the "navel", to foil the dream's attempt to destroy and thus extinguish desire itself. So, we must maintain a distinction between the "Unconscious" (i.e., the repressed which constitutes desire itself) and a "preconscious" or "conscious" wish. *A 'wish' is always a wish to do away with desire (lack) altogether.* We can situate both dream and delusion as

---

[3] I will be referring to this fictional clinical example in this chapter as well as in Chap. 6 on Ethics. Although fictional, this clinical example is relevant in that it retains fundamental and generalizable truths of the psychotic experience and of the logic of treatment. In this chapter the clinical example serves to illustrate key points regarding the logic of dream language versus the language of delusion. In Chap. 6, key clinical moments are highlighted to explore how the *subject* of psychosis can challenge the certainty of delusional certainty.

methods that strive for wish fulfilment; however, the dream is a method that necessarily fails and thus sustains or, as in the case of psychosis, introduces desire.

4.2.4 The Wish Versus Desire: A Wish Aims to Satisfy (Destroy) the [Un]Conscious

By way of delusion, the psychotic travels much further than the neurotic on the path of wish fulfilment—what Freud terms the "path … from excitation [drive] to perception [as satisfaction through hallucination]". In Chap. 2, regarding the psychotic's relation to the lost object of satisfaction, we discussed the following passage from *The Interpretation of Dreams*. Here, this passage is relevant to understanding the relation of the wish to the "motive force" of the dream as "continuous" and "indestructible". Freud (1900) writes:

> [T]he situation [somatic need] remains unaltered, for the excitation arising from an internal need is not due to a force producing a momentary impact but to one which is a continuous operation. (p. 565)

We recognize the "force" that is in "continuous operation" as the insistence of the drive and its cause—the lost object. Freud continues:

> A change can only come about if in some way or other (in the case of a baby, through outside help) an 'experience of satisfaction' can be achieved which puts an end to the internal stimulus. An essential component of this experience of satisfaction is a particular perception … the mnemic image of which remains associated thenceforward with the memory trace of the excitation produced by the need. As a result of the link that has thus been established, next time this need arises a psychical impulse will at once emerge which will seek to re-cathect the mnemic image of the perception and to re-evoke the perception itself, that is to say, to re-establish the situation of the original satisfaction. (p. 565)

The "original satisfaction" to be re-established is equal to the lost object that, in neurosis, constitutes a region of the 'psyche' that is formed by the installation of repression and the Name-of-the-Father, thus symbolizing and stabilizing the effect of the "Un" (the cut, or trauma) that creates the 'Unconscious proper'; something "inadmissible". For the psychotic, we might say that there is indeed a 'loss' but the truth of the loss is, by contrast, admissible to consciousness and thus unbearable, i.e., without representation and therefore experienced in the Real of the body.

So, the specific status of the "motive force" as the cause of the dream and the loss of satisfaction are contingent. For the psychotic the motive force (the "Un") is not repressed or represented. This contingency will be our guide in answering the question regarding the difference between delusion and dream, and why the dream ultimately challenges delusion. Where the neurotic answers the trauma of Language with repression, the Ideals of the Ego, and fantasy, the psychotic chooses "foreclosure" and delusion to explain, and recapture, the radical loss of satisfaction. In Chap. 3, I argued that the psychotic reaches an impasse in transference precisely because of the non-existence of the "inadmissible" (the impossible) and, by extension, the non-existence of symbolic castration. For both Freud and Lacan, the precondition for transference, which for the neurotic hinges upon the supposition of knowledge to the analyst, is primary repression guaranteed by the Name-of-the-Father. The distinction between the existence of symbolic castration (desire) and the experience of the trauma of Language itself is relevant here. It is the existence of symbolic castration (its "representative") that separates neurosis from psychosis. This premise supposes, however, only the 'experience of the trauma of Language' to be universal, i.e., it is the "justification" for the loss of the "original satisfaction" that is in question according to psychical structure.

In the dream, the neurotic wishes for something they imagine themselves to have lost. But the neurotic must be "content", as Freud says, with the compromise offered by the dream. Freud writes: "The infantile scene is unable to bring about its own revival and has to be content with returning as a dream" (p. 546). However, it is more consistent with the psychotic's path to say, as I suggested earlier, that a 'wish' is for the death of desire itself, a wish that (in neurosis) is rendered impossible because of the indestructible (symbolic) barrier between the Unconscious proper and the *Pcs.* and *Cs.* systems.

For the psychotic, the hallucinatory satisfaction provided by the dream is sustained in waking life by delusion. Freud (1900) continues:

> An impulse [for satisfaction] of this kind we call a wish; the reappearance of the perception is the fulfillment of the wish; and the shortest path to the fulfillment of the wish is a path leading direct from the excitation produced by the need to a complete cathexis of the perception. (pp. 565–566)

Here Freud articulates the logic of satisfaction vis-à-vis the path of the "wish", beginning with the "continuous operation" of drive and culminating with the function of the "perceptual identity". Hallucination (the "perceptual identity") is the re-evocation of the perception of the satisfaction of need.

> Nothing prevents us from assuming that there was a primitive state of the psychical apparatus in which this path [from excitation to perception] was actually traversed, that is, in which wishing ended in hallucinating. Thus the aim of this first psychical activity was to produce a 'perceptual identity'—a repetition of the perception which was linked with the satisfaction of the need. (pp. 565–566)

Again, for any subject, the "first psychical activity" implies the consequences, the effects, of the experience of the trauma and the loss of the Real. Finally, later in this same text Freud observes the following:

> The first wishing seems to have been a hallucinatory cathecting of the memory of satisfaction. Such hallucinations, however, if they were not to be maintained *to the point of exhaustion*, proved to be inadequate to bring about the cessation of the need or, accordingly, the pleasure attaching to satisfaction. (italics added, p. 598)

The wish proves "inadequate" to put an end to the "need" in the organism or, subsequently, to achieve the "pleasure attaching to the satisfaction [of the drive]". For the neurotic, the wish fails and she accepts this failure and the series of 'compromises' that follow. However, in psychosis, wishing (hallucination) is indeed maintained "to the point of exhaustion".

The psychotic maintains her wish to be satisfied (her delusion), and to satisfy an Imaginary Other whose demand for jouissance is unlimited.

We might consider the question of "exhaustion" in terms of the exhaustion, or the extinguishing, of desire and thus the exhaustion of the very possibility of a subject for desire. The neurotic, at an earlier point in her subjective history, sacrificed the "first wishing" and thus settled for the symptom, dream, and fantasy as modes of a mediated access to the object. The psychotic, by contrast, clings to, in Freud's words, the moment in the psychical development of the subject at which the "path [from excitation to perception] was actually traversed, i.e., in which wishing ended in hallucinating".

Furthermore, the exhaustion can be witnessed in the psychotic's physical exhaustion where the body is ravaged by the violence of the phenomenology, for example, evidenced in the impossibility of sleep or other basic daily living activities due to a constant fear of annihilation and the compulsion to carry out orders issued by an omnipotent Other. In the clinical example mentioned earlier, an omnipotent Other (represented for him by the "evil voices" and an entity he termed the "Circle of Supreme Beings") compels the subject to annihilate itself both through constant death threats and the requirement for the patient to forgo all creative activities that might provide access to desire. He was prohibited from engaging in his preferred creative endeavour by the "evil voices", i.e., the voices threatened him and his family with death if he chose to defy the prohibition. For this person, the Other's desire is rendered as a pure Demand, or "wish", to destroy the subject and desire itself. The Other's wish is the patient's command.

So the question becomes: How far is the subject willing, or compelled, to go on the path of wish fulfilment? Will the subject settle for the dream as a compromised form of satisfaction, where the object remains impossible, or will the subject insist upon total satisfaction as in the case of the psychotic and her delusion? With the psychotic's delusion we have a "complete cathexis" of a "perception" (e.g., voice and delusion) that constitutes, as Freud terms it, the "shortest path to the fulfillment of the wish"—a wish that is, by definition, against desire.

4.3 The Law of Dream Language and the Introduction of Desire Itself

4.3.1 Dream Introduces a New Opposition Into the Psychical Life of the Psychotic

The dream is opposed to delusion insofar as the dream functions according to the laws of language whereas delusion does not. The opposition is in fact between different knowledges—different structures, for example a linguistic structure that is lacking (dream) versus a structure, or universe, without lack (delusion). The "laws" of dream language, following Freud, are condensation and displacement, or what Lacan later termed metaphor and metonymy respectively. Psychoanalyst Lucie Cantin (2002) writes: "To each [dream] image must be given back the word, the formula, the proverb that the dream image sets up" (p. 88). Of course the "image" to which the "word", the interpretation, must be offered, is an image conjured by the Real. Cantin continues: "Thus, the interpretation of the dream reveals the laws that govern its elaboration" (p. 88). In the dream, evidenced in the "laws that govern its elaboration", there exists a lack between the Real, as radically lost, and the representation that ultimately fails to represent it. As Cantin formulates it, the dream attempts "to treat the Real with something symbolic" (p. 87). Thus, the term "law", regarding the dream, implies an internal limit to language, insofar as language, because it may only strive to re-present the "thing", is fundamentally lacking and thus constitutes a desiring structure, versus a complete knowledge as found in delusion. It is in this sense of an internal limit to dream language that, previously, I have referred to the 'dream's castration'.

It is often repeated, perhaps without understanding why, that for the psychotic 'words are things'. In delusion, we can hear evidence of the collapse of the distinction between word and thing, yet we must be careful to observe that the collapse is not simply between any word and any thing, but between the Word (a primary [paternal] metaphor) and the maternal "Thing" (as in one's access to complete satisfaction or jouissance). For example, in the patient's delusion, the "Circle of Supreme

Beings" does not represent any[thing] or anyone else, but instead occupies the status of an absolute Other subject to no law but their own. As the patient says in response to my inquiry, there is the possibility that the "Supreme Beings" may limit the influence and power of the "evil voices", yet "no one [no law/limit] controls the Supreme Beings". So, we might say that, by definition, delusion is 'lawless'.

By contrast, the patient's dreams lead to associations and memories that, in turn, produce a series of little others (e.g., the patient's "father", his "supervisor", and "older brother"). I refer the reader to Chap. 6 on Ethics for further elaboration of this latter point. However, in brief, I argue that the 'little others' introduced by the dream function to figure the patient's relation to 'authority' and by extension to the Law and the failure of the paternal metaphor itself.

4.3.2 The Dream Evokes a "Subjective History" which Contests Delusion

As the clinical example indicates, the dream evokes memories that, for the psychotic under transference, come to represent the subject's relation to lack and to the Law. Where the delusion functions to refuse lack, the dream and its failure (re)introduces lack, both as trauma and, potentially, as cause of desire. Psychoanalyst Danielle Bergeron (2002) writes of the confrontation of dream with delusion:

> The interest of the dream with the psychotic ... consists in the fact that, through the signifiers, a *savoir* of the unconscious—in the form of fragments of the signifying chain [associative material] encircling a hole—is substituted for the dense certitude of delusion and for the delusionary knowledge that blocks any representation of lack. (p. 77)

However, the possibility of substituting an "unconscious savoir" for the "certitude of delusion" raises a question about the status of the dream and the time of its emergence under transference. For example, the first dreams produced by the psychotic do not always function according to the 'law of lanaguage', and thus fail to oppose delusion with lack. Lucie

Cantin explains that it is often the case that the first dreams produced by the psychotic patient are "indistiguishable from the logic of delusion, which they more or less reproduce" (p. 98). The psychotic may offer a dream that produces associations that, rather than lead to memories, link directly to the content and logic of delusion. The mark of a 'real' dream is found in the nature of the associations produced by the dream. A 'real' dream, what we term a true "psychoanalytic dream", must evoke childhood memories and traumatic events that lead the psychotic towards elements of his "subjective" (singular) history of encounters with the Real and with the threat of castration.

For example, the dream(s) evoke a series of memories which, in the course of treatment, begin to construct a 'history' of the subject's encounter with, and failure of, symbolic castration. So, we might say that the dream evokes the traumatic history of the subject that the delusion, thus far, had attempted to 'theorize'. In Chap. 6 the reader will see precisely how the analyst's desire (evidenced in the questioning of the dream's content) leads the patient to discover elements of his subjective history which function, ultimately, to pierce a hole in the certainty of his delusion.

4.4 The Stakes of the Choice of the Dream, and Its Law, Given the Foreclosure of the Name-of-the-Father

4.4.1 The Lack of a "Lacking Signifier"

Returning to Bergeron's remarks, the signifying chain is "substituted" for the "certitude of delusion". There is an interesting conflation here of the content and the form of the dream. A question emerges regarding the difference between the substitution of content (memories etc.) versus the introduction of the mechanism of substitution (metonymy) itself. The difference between 'substitution itself' and the substitution of memory content is crucial to understanding the status of the dream in psychosis and, furthermore, this difference is the key to locating how the dream introduces castration and desire itself. With the psychotic, the dream, when it is evoked by the analyst's desire, introduces a new form: a new, ever-shifting, and incomplete structure of knowledge.

Bergeron (2002) illuminates a key distinction between the functioning of the dream in neurosis versus psychosis: in neurosis, the movement of the dream-work is from "signifier to signifier, encircling the real ['navel'], and progressively symbolizing the untold moments of the analysand's life" (p. 77). Bergeron continues:

> With the neurotic, the very structure of the dream chains the signifiers around a *lacking signifier*, that unacknowledged thing in the navel of the dream. With the psychotic, by contrast, the signifiers may reorganize but will not fully chain. It is rather the analyst's maneuver that directs these segments of signifying chain to an inevitable confrontation with whatever in the psychotic's history has remained without representation. (italics added, pp. 77–78)

In neurosis, the Name-of-the-Father is the "lacking signifier" but it is a signifier nonetheless—that is, a signifier that, by repressing the Void, creates the conditions for the articulation and metaphorization of lack. Note, in addition, that "the very structure of the dream", as Bergeron phrases it, is determined by the status of the "motive force (cause) and the functioning of the "navel" as the limit point of representation in the dream. The structure, or structuring, of the dream by 'lack' in this way is specific to neurosis. The signifiers of the dream, in neurosis, chain (collect) around the void in knowledge that is repressed by the Name-of-the-Father. Yet, it would seem that the chaining is facilitated by the Name-of-the-Father and not the Void, insofar as the Name-of-the-Father is required for any chaining, or articulation, whatsoever.

Thus, by contrast, we can posit that in psychosis the signifiers do not "fully chain" because of the absence of the Name-of-the-Father and, therefore, the failure of a master signifier (S1) to set the signifying chain in motion. In other words, in psychosis there exists no lost 'One', as signified by the Name-of-the-Father in neurosis, to cause the metonymic movement from signifier to signifier in search of an irrevocably lost signifier. Yet it is the metonymic and metaphorical function of the dream language that challenges delusion and reintroduces the effects of castration. If the lawful function of language is absent in psychotic structure, then how (by what method) will the psychotic be guided to encounter the limit of language in the dream? In other words, what sustains the psychotic subject in the face of the void opened up by the dream and, more to the point, what supports the subject where the Name-of-the-Father (as "lacking signifier" in neurosis) is itself non-lacking or, in other words, foreclosed?

4.4.2 The Analyst's "Manoeuvre" in the Place of the 'Object a'

The analyst "maneuvers" from the position of the 'object a' and thus, in the case of psychosis, from a contestatory position vis-à-vis delusion. In the early phase of treatment, Bergeron writes, the analyst—in the place of the 'object a'—functions as a "support" for the subject where the dream tears a hole in delusion, thus confronting the subject with its trauma as 'cause'. But, we might ask, what supports this "support"? Bergeron says that in psychosis it is the analyst's manoeuvre that will direct the unchained signifying elements (memory fragments) towards an "inevitable confrontation with whatever in the psychotic's [subjective] history has remained without representation". In other words, the analyst's manoeuvre will direct the "signifying [lacking/desiring] elements" towards delusion. Now, Lacan himself taught that the analyst acts from the position of the 'object a', and Lacan's teaching on this point did not pertain to the treatment of psychotics but in the direction, primarily, of the analytic treatment of neurotics. If the analyst acts from the position of the lost object of desire regardless of psychical structure, then what, precisely, is implied by the careful distinction made by Bergeron regarding the analyst's "maneuver" in psychosis?

The distinction regards the unique status of the 'object a' in psychosis and its bearing on the position required by the analyst: the analyst's desire functions differently in the encounter with psychosis than with neurosis. In psychosis, it is the analyst's desire, which supposes the very *possibility* of lack, that functions as a support in the "confrontation" between "segments of the signifying chain" and "whatever in the psychotic's history has remained without representation". Bergeron's notion of the analyst's desire as "support" follows Apollon's (1991) thesis that the psychotic, under transference, responds to the analyst's desire as support by, ultimately, constructing an object that functions as a "surrogate for the lack of the signifier of the Father" (p. 138). Apollon writes:

> The object [constructed by the psychotic analysand] arrives at the place where the analyst stood for the object a, solely by his presence, framing the void opened by the foreclosure of the signifier of the Father. (p. 138)

The key point here is that, for the psychotic, there will arise, in the course of treatment, a moment where the subject may choose to confront the defect in Language without the delusion, but also without the Name-of-the-Father and, by extension, the illusion provided by the Ideals of the Ego. Bergeron (2002) writes: "The analyst in the position of the object *a* is necessarily the link between the chain segments and the real in … psychosis" (p. 78). It is not the analyst per se, but the analyst's desire vis-à-vis the 'object a' 'in' him or her (the analyst) that functions as the "link" (and as the 'limit') that articulates the failure of delusion and its consequences for the subject <u>to</u> the structural defect in Language. This is saying quite a lot, given the status of the 'defect' for the psychotic. This last claim supports the following thesis regarding the future of the psychotic under transference: the structural defect in Language, a purely formal question, is faced by the psychotic after the delusion begins to fall but, under transference, with the analyst's desire as a temporary barrier between the subject and the horror of the Void.

The psychotic's confrontation with the defect in Language under transference brings forth a question regarding the function of *ethics* that I will only pose here: If the functioning of the analyst's desire is temporary, can the subject that ultimately confronts the defect in language (the subject alone without illusion) be the same subject as that which chose foreclosure and, ultimately, delusion? It is as though the contestation, the "rupture", of delusion by the dream creates the conditions for a 'second choice' in the face of the rupture, or 'event', that marks the emergence of desire itself. In other words, is this not a subject (she who has encountered the loss of delusion) that has found, again, the possibility of a choice, thus signalling a shift in position, the precondition for which is the production of a new ethics?

Given the foreclosure of the Name-of-the-Father, Willy Apollon suggests an ultimate possibility for the psychotic who reaches the conclusion of analysis. He writes:

> Thenceforth, at the end of the [treatment] process the psychotic subject finds herself at the starting point facing the want in the Other, *without* the support of a still lacking signifier. (italics mine, p. 139)

Without the "still lacking signifier", in other words the Name-of-the-Father, the psychotic subject must face the Void without any neurotic illusion or psychotic certainty. Apollon continues:

> [S]he is no longer in the position of looking for a final truth in the foundation of the world … she has experienced the division that language introduces into mankind as a structural one and not as an evil whose responsible party she has to identify. (p. 139)

Apollon's conclusion, that the psychotic ultimately, under transference, accepts castration without the fundamental libidinal tie afforded to the neurotic, opens the way to a discussion of ethics in the forthcoming chapter: an ethics without recourse to the Good (Ideals) or to the certitude of delusion.

The "link" provided by the analyst's desire 'stands in' for lack itself insofar as, in psychosis, the analyst's desire is the only desire in play—I contend—prior to the emergence of the dream and transference. The analyst, in his or her 'act', seems to convey the following to the psychotic: "Yes there exists something lost (the 'object a') and the [analyst's] insistence upon desire [originating from the dream] attests to this 'fact' as the precondition, and possibility, for you to take the place of a desiring subject."

4.4.3 The Psychotic's Savoir and the Analyst's Hypothesis

Given the specific status of the 'object a' in psychosis, Bergeron suggests such a contestatory function for the analyst's desire in the treatment of psychosis:

> At the place of the impossible object of desire, the object *a*, the analyst contests the position of the psychotic as object of the jouissance of the Other. (p. 78)

However, as I have argued, this "place of the impossible object" is non-existent in the psychotic's universe and, although the 'object a' is a fact of the analyst's experience and desire, it is maintained at the level of a mere hypothesis *for* the psychotic *by* the analyst. We must not forget that the psychotic's *savoir* regards the 'senseless' defect in Language and, furthermore, that the delusion is only a theory of the psychotic's *savoir.* Cantin (2002) writes that with psychotics "the problem lies not with the knowledge itself, but with the fact that the *savoir* [via delusion] aims at being complete and flawless" (p. 95). There is an implied distinction here between the psychotic's "*savoir*", regarding the defect, and the "aim" with which the psychotic takes the *savoir* in the field of delusion towards a "[f]lawless" solution for the defect in Language. It is only by maintaining the distinction between the analyst's hypothesis and the psychotic's "*savoir*" that we may comprehend the true stakes for the psychotic in the movement from delusion to dream (from the Real to representation).

4.5 The Function of the Dream in the Installation and "Reversal" of Transference

Here I provide a general introduction to the concept of the reversal of the analyst's position in the field of psychosis versus neurosis. It is important for the reader to grasp the stakes for, and responsibility of, the analyst in the encounter with the psychotic's delusion and in the face of what Freud termed the psychotic's "indifference". It is the mishandling of the psychotic's seeming indifference (a lack of a desire to know) that can lead to a botched encounter with the psychotic.

4.5.1 The Analyst's Position in the Neurotic Dialectic

Danielle Bergeron, in a lecture entitled "Transference: From the Patient's Demand to the Analysand's Responsibility" (2003),[4] has stated that

> the patient arrives with a demand for love. But, the analyst is always in the position of the one who lacks, who doesn't know. This position will provoke in him [the patient], unconscious productions.

First, it should be noted that in this quote Bergeron is referring to the stakes of transference in treating neurosis, hence the author's reference to the elements of the seduction fantasy (demand for love and completeness) typically in play in the neurotic transference. In the field of neurosis, the analyst is met by a patient with a "demand for love". We can think of this demand, also, as a demand for knowledge from the one who is "supposed to know", namely the analyst. The neurotic patient loves and hates the analyst precisely because the analyst 'knows'. So, with neurosis, the analyst is in the position of the one who is supposed to know the truth, or cause, that perpetuates the suffering of the subject.

In the fantasy of the neurotic patient who makes a demand for love, the analyst is the 'one' who holds the key to the subject's desire. The analyst meets the demand of the patient with a desire to know, and thus introduces a lack that confronts the patient's demand for love and completion with a question aimed at the subject of the unconscious. The interface of the demand for love and the analyst's desire introduces the first "reversal" of transference as it occurs in the field of neurosis. The reversal implies that the knowledge required to provide a choice to the

[4] Bergeron, D. (2003, June). *Transference: From the patient's demand to the analysand's Responsibility*. Lecture delivered in the context of the "Annual Training Seminar in Lacanian Psychoanalysis". Quebec City, Canada.

analysand is supposed to be on the side of the subject of the unconscious, not *in* the analyst. In short, the analyst must 'de-suppose' him or herself and, as Bergeron following Lacan's notes, assume the position of the one who lacks (knowledge).

4.5.2 The "Reversal" of the Analytic Position with the Psychotic

In the field of psychosis the stakes of the reversal differ dramatically from those of neurosis. Where the neurotic doubts, and thus supposes the analyst to know, the psychotic knows with great certainty and therefore does not position the analyst in the address as the one supposed to know. We find the primary example of such certainty in the form and content of the psychotic's delusion. As defined earlier, the function of the delusion in psychosis is first to theorize, and second to provide a solution for the suffering inherent in the psychotic experience of the Void. The delusion functions to "explain" and to "justify" the psychotic's experience of a subjection to an all-powerful and abusive Other. Key, however, is that the "delusion is not simply an explanatory effort; it is also a tentative solution, an attempt to escape from the position of being the object of the jouissance [omnipotence/abuse] of the Other" (Cantin, p. 92). The shift from explanation to 'solution' marks a shift, for the psychotic, from an object of abuse to an agent in the scheme of the delusion. With the patient mentioned earlier, we witness the shift from object to agent, that is internal to delusion, in his affirmation of the impossible demands placed upon him to be, as the patient says, a "Nobel Laureate".

However, the movement from object of the jouissance of the Other to the position of an 'agent in the delusion' must be distinguished from the movement from 'delusion to dream'. As noted earlier, the movement from delusion to dream marks the emergence of the space of desire, and of the subject. The movement from delusion to dream requires a shift that constitutes, if risked, a change in the subject's relation to jouissance, and a potential opening of the space of desire-as-barrier to jouissance.

We can suppose that the stakes of the dream follow from Cantin's premise which states that "the dream implies a breach [rupture] of that knowledge, that 'savoir'" that the analyst must suppose to the delusion, and thus suppose to the psychotic. The 'stakes' introduced by the dream, then, involve the potential loss of delusion or, more to the point, a confrontation with the radical loss that delusion attempts to satisfy (treat) once and for all. Therefore, to provoke the transference in the field of psychosis, the analyst must 'suppose the psychotic to know', thus reversing the usual analytic positions in which the neurotic supposes the analyst to know and enters the affective transference via a demand for love.

The attribution of knowing to the psychotic requires that the analyst hold the conviction that there exists in the delusion a specific knowledge about the advent of a given subject. This conviction, which supposes a knowing subject to the psychotic experience, functions as the basis of the analyst's ethic, and sustains the analyst's desire in the face of pure delusion, or, in other words, prior to the time in treatment where the dream emerges to challenge the certainty of delusion. The specific knowledge in the delusion, fundamentally, regards the rupture, or "break-in", of Language and the "voice" into the fullness of the organism and the inadequacy of the signifier to provide a limit to the Other's Demand for jouissance.

In the patient's discourse we can hear the "Demands" of the "Supreme Beings" as representative of an uncastrated Other that possesses absolute rule over the patient's experience. Again, the subject of the unconscious finds its cause in the moment of the "break-in" of the Other of Language and, thus, the subject has inscribed in its body a knowledge or "*savoir*" concerning the experience of rupture (as cause). It is the cause (as "rupture") that the dream, ultimately, evokes which in turn challenges delusion, thus providing the psychotic with a choice of dream versus delusion, or of desire versus satisfaction respectively.

The question of the psychotic's certainty, then, brings forth the specific question of the "reversal" of the usual analytic position. The term reversal refers to the analyst's position vis-à-vis the delusion itself and, in addition, to the question of how (by what method) to contest the delusion's certainty. The analyst must position him or herself such that "it is the psychotic subject, not the analyst, who takes the position of the one 'supposed to know'" (Cantin, p. 95). Yet, for the purpose of this argument, I want to modify Cantin's observation to emphasize precisely how difficult the shift from delusion to dream actually is. I suggest that the subject itself (its very existence) must be supposed, and that is precisely what the analyst does, i.e., the analyst maintains the hypothesis that there is a subject *of* the knowledge we call delusion. This distinction suggests two separate aspects of the said reversal of the analytic positions. In addition, supposing the existence of the subject itself follows from the earlier formulation, 'castration (as cause of the subject) is a mere hypothesis of the analyst'. In other words, at the beginning of the treatment, the analyst is alone with a desire to know in the face of delusion. Maintaining the distinction (supposing the subject 'to know' versus supposing the subject 'itself') is relevant because it underscores the true stakes for the psychotic in the choice of desire and castration (dream) over certainty (delusion), and the stakes for the analyst who is alone in the face of delusion with only his or her conviction to guide the way.

So, there are two "reversals", one on the side of the analyst, and a second required by the psychotic—a reversal evidenced by the emergence of the dream and a commitment to pursuing the dream-work. It is the reversal on the side of the psychotic that signals the installation of transference—transference as desire itself, and as a desire to know.

The first reversal regards the analyst's position prior to the emergence of the dream, i.e., in the face of pure delusion. We can see an example of this 'first' reversal in the case noted earlier. For example, in the beginning of the treatment the patient's discourse consisted entirely of delusion, and the analyst's position functioned to suppose a subject of (1) her system of disturbing beliefs (delusion) and (2) the traumatic encounter with the Other (and little others) that the delusion theorizes. The second reversal regards the relation of the psychotic analysand to her own unconscious structure (e.g., including its productions). This reversal supposes two things however: the emergence of the subject as such, and a continued work under transference to follow the subject of the unconscious in the effort to construct a new knowledge that will ultimately undermine the utility of delusion. The dream is required for the second reversal on the side of the psychotic analysand, and it is the question of the second reversal that is raised in the clinical discussion in Chap. 6 on ethics.

4.6 Conclusion: The Choice of the Dream

It is the dream, its lacking (and 'lawful') structure, that, paradoxically, evokes the structural defect in Language and the Law, thus challenging the certitude of delusion, yet, and this is key, without obliterating the psychotic's *savoir*. The moment when the analyst's desire "contests" the position of the psychotic as "object of the *jouissance* of the Other", he creates the conditions for a new choice for the psychotic, and clarifies the stakes for the psychotic in the face of a new choice either to remain in the field of delusion or enter transference and follow the letter. The question of the subject's shift in relation to the body of the letter, and to death drive, brings us to the problem of "ethics" as that which is produced in a moment of rupture, and in the moment of the subject's shift, or choice, vis-à-vis the surging forth of drive.

References

Apollon, W. (1991). Theory and practice in the psychoanalytic practice of psyhosis. In E. Ragland-Sullivan & M. Bracher (Eds.), *Lacan and the subject of language* (pp. 116–140). Routledge.

Bergeron, D. (2002). The work of the dream and jouissance in the treatment of the psychotic. In R. Hughes & K. R. Malone (Eds.), *After Lacan: Clinical practice and the subject of the unconscious* (pp. 71–85). SUNY Press.

Cantin, L. (2002). From delusion to dream. In R. Hughes & K. R. Malone (Eds.), *After Lacan: Clinical practice and the subject of the unconscious* (pp. 87–102). SUNY Press.

Freud, S. (1900). *The interpretation of dreams.* SE Vols. IV&V, 1999.

5

The Utility of Gilles Deleuze's Critique of Psychoanalysis

5.1 Preliminary to a Discussion of Ethics

In siding with the psychotic, Deleuze and Guattari raise questions that cause psychoanalysis to re-examine its most basic precepts and, furthermore, to clarify what is most compelling about Lacan's *savoir*, namely the subject's relation to the object, and to death drive as the possible locus of ethics.

Deleuze and Guattari charge that psychoanalysis "botches the encounter with the psychotic", and ultimately with the Real. Deleuze and Guattari offer an ethics (a "program", a "set of practices"), but one that is ostensibly free of and from the Law and castration. Of course Lacan argues for an ethics that is 'against' the Law (as pure command), but it is an ethics in relation to the Law, and to castration, nonetheless. I will argue that (1) the said distinction between Deleuze and Guattari and Lacan is founded on a typical misreading of Deleuze and Guattari regarding the function of the Law and by contrast (2) that Deleuze and Guattari in fact follow Lacan on the question of the body and of desire and, ultimately, support our effort to construct an ethics derived from the psychotic's savoir of the Law.

B. Fimiani, *Psychosis and Extreme States*, The Palgrave Lacan Series,
https://doi.org/10.1007/978-3-030-75440-2_5

5.2 The Lost Body of the Psychotic as the "Body without Organs" of Psychoanalysis

> Psychoanalysis is like capitalism: although it tends toward the limit of schizophrenia, it's constantly evading this limit, and trying to get around it. (Deleuze, *Negotiations*, 1995, p. 21)

Deleuze's claim, that psychoanalysis "has no way of facing schizophrenia directly", rests on the premise that psychoanalysis is a fundamentally repressive force that resituates all experience, all "desiring production", in the domestic (read Oedipalizing) versus the social field:

> [Psychoanalysis] neuroticizes everything, and through this neuroticization contributes not only to producing neurotics whose treatment never ends but also psychotics in the form of anyone resisting oedipalization.

In this quote Deleuze locates a main hazard (and question) for psychoanalysis in the face of psychosis: Does psychoanalysis avoid the truth of psychosis by viewing the phenomenon of psychosis through a neurotic lens? Deleuze's claim, however, which dismisses psychoanalysis categorically, becomes problematic when considered more closely in terms of Lacan's reformulation of Oedipus, and Lacan's discovery regarding the status of knowledge in the field of psychosis. What is in question here is the ethic of the analyst. I will define and discuss ethics at length in the following chapter. A preview should suffice for this discussion: ethics implies that the analyst will not attempt to deploy consensual or neurotic knowledge(s) to understand the psychotic. Instead, an ethical approach to treating psychosis requires that the psychotic be met on their own terms. This would render the imposition by the analyst of a neurotic knowledge (or epistemology) to engage the psychotic inherently unethical.

5.2.1 The Body and Ethics

It is important not to lose sight of the connection between the body and ethics. Deleuze and Guattari, following Lacan, isolate the body as the contestatory, and thus the guiding force that is key in locating the subject. Deleuze and Guattari (with Lacan) open the way to a thorough interrogation of two questions central to the linkage between the body and ethics:

1. How does psychosis—which implicates the body in psychical structure—constitute a limit for psychoanalysis itself? [1]
2. What are the implications for psychoanalysis as a praxis in the confrontation with psychosis as a field of contestation, or limit? And, by extension, how can psychoanalysis avoid, as Deleuze and Guattari put it, "botching the real" of the body?

I have designated two possible, and distinct, choices made by the subject of psychosis regarding the confrontation with the Void, and the excess (jouissance) introduced by Language. The first choice concerns what Lacan terms a "forced choice" in the moment of the subjection of the organism to Language and the Ideals of society. The second choice concerns the choice based for the subject on the analyst's offering to enter into symbolic exchange and the economy of desire. In psychoanalysis, we locate the second choice, which can only take place under transference, as a choice that initiates and grounds the subject's creation of a new ethic.

I will articulate the conceptual linkage between Lacan, and Deleuze and Guattari regarding the status of the body as a contestatory force. Following Lacan and Freud, the body is on the side of the lost object, and so the body is itself a lost body—a body that contests precisely because it is a body constituted in, and by, its resistance to the organizing function of signification and the phallus. Deleuze and Guattari (1983, 1987) are instructive regarding the question of the body and the body's function as site of contestation.

---

[1] As discussed in Chap. 3, for both Freud and Lacan psychosis represented a subjective (and clinical) field that led to an impasse under transference.

First, we must confront the impasse that arises in the attempt to interface Deleuze and Guattari, and Lacan. It should be understood, as preliminary to what follows, that when Deleuze and Guattari refer to "schizophrenia" the authors make a distinction between the "clinical" and the "experimental" relation to the experience of schizophrenia or psychosis. For Deleuze and Guattari, it is not a question of clinical 'treatment' but of what Deleuze terms in *Dialogues* (1987) a process of "extraction". The point, following Deleuze and Guattari, is to experiment with, and to extract from certain experiences (e.g., psychosis, addiction), the "lines of flight" and "becomings" that they offer, not to bog down, the authors warn, in the experience or "practice" and become an "empty" ("catatonicized") "non-desiring" body. Consequently, for Deleuze and Guattari, schizophrenia as a "process" or "program" (versus a destination or 'clinical state') either succeeds in creating a "desiring body that works" or fails. It is the psychoanalyst, on the other hand, who is interested in the 'failure to desire' that is characteristic of 'psychosis-as-clinical-state'.

Deleuze and Guattari's interrogation of psychoanalysis is important precisely because it locates what is truly at stake for the subject (e.g., the Real as contestatory), even though their critique fails to apprehend accurately the nature of the "Oedipal Law" as elaborated and deployed by Lacan. For example, Lacan's primary innovation was to posit a *savoir*, a specific knowledge, and thus the possibility of an ethic beyond Oedipus and thus beyond the guarantee for an Ideal. Deleuze and Guattari locate the status of the subject with a conception of the body (i.e., "Body without Organs") as a limit to structure and organization. Thus, even with Deleuze and Guattari, we have an empty function represented by the Body without Organs that serves to delimit the space of the subject, or lost body-as-letter, that is key for our understanding of what is at stake in the treatment of psychosis.

I contend that Deleuze and Guattari, contrary to the typical reading of *Anti-Oedipus* and *A Thousand Plateaus*, do not succeed in making a full departure from the fundamental premise of psychoanalysis. For now, we can say that psychoanalysis, as a praxis, rests upon the premise that the subject and desire are caused by the effect of the Law, and it is not a question of reinstituting an 'authoritarian', or "Oedipalizing" (as Deleuze and Guattari would have it), psychoanalysis. The typical reading of Deleuze and Guattari's argument regarding psychoanalysis situates Deleuze and Guattari against Lacan, and Freud, regarding the question of desire, and the status of the Law of lack as cause of desire. The usual opposition requires that, for Lacan, desire is lack and that, for Deleuze and Guattari, desire is a purely positive force lacking nothing. For this study, we are interested in where this dichotomy 'lack/fullness' breaks down. In particular, Deleuze and Guattari's attempt to render desire without lack runs aground (1) regarding the question of "organism/body" opposition, and (2) regarding their equating of the figure of Oedipus, and thus repression, with the position of the analyst. For Deleuze and Guattari, the psychotic always and already has an ethic vis-à-vis death drive that requires no intervention, the authors argue, by the methods of psychoanalysis—as Deleuze and Guattari say, "[a] psychotic out for a walk is a better model than the neurotic lying on the analyst's couch" (*Anti-Oedipus*, 1983, p. 2).

5.2.2 The Body as Limit in Deleuze and Guattari, and Lacan

What is the body for Deleuze and Guattari? Thus far we have situated the body as letter, following Lacan, in opposition to the organism. However, it appears that Deleuze and Guattari's use of the term "organism" differs substantially from that of Lacan. This brings us to the first problem with Deleuze and Guattari's critique. From the standpoint of psychoanalysis, the fullness of organism is posited in order to designate the category of the impossible for the speaking being. The Law is the mark that separates the possible and impossible, and subsequently institutes the dialectic of the full versus the empty, or jouissance and desire respectively.

Psychoanalysis, as a praxis, cannot function without the basic premise of a fundamental lack that indicates a prior fantasized fullness or totality. Lacan's deployment of the term "organism" implies the full, uncut by language, biological entity, e.g., the animal that functions according to an instinct with a prescribed object of satisfaction. But for Lacan it is only a logical necessity of neurosis to posit a state prior to the trauma of language—a state to which we have no access, except, as Freud tells us, through its "representatives". In other words, to understand the logic of neurosis (its phenomenology of fantasy, guilt, and depression), psychoanalysis concedes to the neurotic the illusion of a lost fullness or 'Paradise'. This is the basis, as well, for the stability of castration as a concept in psychoanalysis—the experience of castration, and anguish, under transference is, for the neurotic, set against (requires) the retrospective illusion of a lost Paradise. It is precisely this distinction (that is fundamental to psychoanalysis) between lack and fullness, a distinction installed by prohibition and repression, that Deleuze and Guattari take issue with.

For Deleuze and Guattari, the distinction of 'organism/body' requires no reference to a prohibited jouissance, such that the 'organism', as Deleuze and Guattari use the term, is already the product of social forces. Deleuze and Guattari do not seem to posit a prior state of (imagined/fantasized) full being in the way that Lacan does. Against Lacan, Deleuze and Guattari (1983) write: "The body without organs is not the proof of an original nothingness, nor what remains of a lost totality" (Anti-Oedipus, p. 8). The "lost totality" presupposes a lack as the cause of desire.

However, with the opposition of "Body without Organs/desiring machine" Deleuze and Guattari seem to propose an image of the body as subject to an economy of lack. Deleuze and Guattari invoke the "body without organs" as a site that resists any and all organizing functions, e.g., the Body without Organs versus "desiring machines". Deleuze and Guattari write: "The full body without organs is the unproductive, the sterile, the unengendered, the unconsumable" (p. 8). The body (without organs), then, is what is (must be) produced as "anti-production" to disarticulate the organism that is itself born of socio-libidinal imperatives. Desiring machines, which function in opposition to the Body without Organs, are organizing machines that cut into the "full body".

> Desiring machines make us an organism; but at the very heart of this production, within the very production of this production, the body suffers from being organized in this way, from not having some other sort of organization, or no organization at all. (p. 8)

What is the "body that suffers" here? The body, according to Deleuze and Guattari, suffers from organization itself, or of not being organized otherwise, i.e., the body suffers from "not having some other sort of organization". The body suffers from 'not having'? What do Deleuze and Guattari suggest as the model for libidinal-economy? Is the Body without Organs composed of the 'excess' that is excluded by a given composition of "desiring machines?" This would constitute an economy of lack/desire articulated by Lacan and Freud, and that is proper to psychoanalysis. Or, does the "other sort of organization" presuppose an economy without lack, such that Deleuze and Guattari's 'experimenter' could exchange one totalizing socio-libidinal-economic organization (or composition of desiring machines) for another, one "program" for another? The idea here is that the body suffers because it has no choice regarding its organization, no choice in the apparatuses that organize it, or the effect (i.e., "suffering") of organization itself.

We must also presume that this "other sort of organization" would produce a new 'suffering body', also at a loss, because it does not have something 'other'. The desiring machines, as defined by Deleuze and Guattari, produce one possible expression, or mode of "becoming", for the Body without Organs. But this sounds like desire in the psychoanalytic sense, wherein desire is caused by the gap introduced into, and inherent in, the effect of articulation, or the cut—"*Desiring Machines work only when they break down, and by continually breaking down*" (p. 8). So we have "break down", or desire-as-articulation defined by the limit *represented* by the 'body'. In *A Thousand Plateaus* (1987) the authors write: "[Y]ou never reach the Body without Organs, you can't reach it, you are forever attaining it, it is a limit" (p. 150).

How, and regarding what, does the Body without Organs function as a limit? The authors warn of a too rapid "de-stratification" and suggest "caution" to be the best route to approach the Body without Organs. The Body without Organs presents itself as a limit, beyond which is death.

> Staying stratified—organized, signified, subjected—is not the worst thing that can happen; the worst thing that can happen is if you throw the strata into suicidal collapse, which brings them back down on you heavier than ever. (p. 161)

Psychosis-as-clinical-state, Deleuze and Guattari argue, is the consequence of proceeding with too little 'caution' and in turn "wildly destratifying":

> You have to keep enough of the organism for it to reform each dawn; and you have to keep small supplies of significance and subjectification, if only to turn them against their own systems when the circumstances demand it. ... You don't reach the Body without Organs ... by wildly destratifying. That is why we encountered the paradox of those emptied and dreary [schizophrenic, addicted] bodies at the beginning: *they had emptied themselves of their organs* instead of looking for the point at which they could patiently and momentarily dismantle the organization of the organs we call the organism. (author's italics, pp. 160–161)

So, the Body without Organs constitutes a limit that is "unattainable" and that thus merely 'represents', or corresponds to, the contestation of imposed, or "rigid", structures (e.g., "stratification" in Deleuze and Guattari's terms). In *Anti-Oedipus*, Deleuze and Guattari situate the Body without Organs in terms of death drive, or the "full body" of death:

> The death instinct: that is its name, and death is not without a model. For desire desires death also, because the full body of death is its motor, just as it desires life, because the organs of life are the *working machine.* (p. 8)

With Deleuze and Guattari *we have desire (as composition or cut) functioning as antidote to the full body of death.* The Body without Organs, then, is on the side of death drive. However, Deleuze and Guattari do not explicitly account for the production of the 'body' and death drive by reference to the negativity of Language. Deleuze and Guattari reproach Lacan and Freud for their reliance on death (i.e., symbolic castration) as the fundamental limit in psychoanalysis. The "full body of death", the "full Body without Organs", is unattainable, and therefore evokes the impossible, and the 'necessary loss' required for desire to circulate.

For the purpose of this argument, I contend that Deleuze and Guattari's 'full body' occupies the place of Lacan's usage of "organism" without lack as a representation, or indicator, of the impossible. Transgression of

Deleuze and Guattari's rule, which situates the Body without Organs as unattainable, leads to the possible psychical death of the subject. With both Lacan, and Deleuze and Guattari we have the necessity of founding 'life' on the symbolic death of an imagined fullness. It is the loss of access to drive's full satisfaction, elaborated in Lacan and by Deleuze and Guattari, that forms the castrated subject. Deleuze and Guattari install an opposition between that which produces the 'cut' ("stratification") and that which resists stratification (organization)—the Body without Organs and the Real of the Body. The key is to support the interface of the opposing forces of 'structure' and that which escapes or 'contests'.

5.2.3 Regarding the Position of the Analyst, and Protecting the Psychotic's Savoir

Deleuze and Guattari raise a question that is key to solving a problem at issue in this study: *How do we not "botch" the encounter with the psychotic?* Of course Deleuze and Guattari charge psychoanalysis with precisely this, "botching the Real" in the encounter with the psychotic. Deleuze and Guattari argue, in *Anti-Oedipus* and *A Thousand Plateaus*, that psychoanalysis simply resituates the psychotic on the Oedipal plane, thus stripping the psychotic of the inherent contestatory force of its intimate bodily knowledge regarding the rules of social coexistence as unfounded. I suggest that the difference between Deleuze and Guattari, and Lacan, concerning the problem of the body and social contestation, primarily regards method, rather than a fundamentally different conception of the subject and desire. However much Deleuze and Guattari differ from Lacan in their conception of the proper method to access 'desire' (e.g., "schizoanalysis" versus psychoanalysis), Deleuze and Guattari propose the conception of the 'body' as a site of social contestation) with great clarity.

What is compelling about Deleuze and Guattari's thinking on the phenomenon of psychosis is their emphasis on various "practices" aimed at "experimentation" with the "strata". Note that Deleuze and Guattari's conception of "experimentation" situates the psychotic as one who is actively engaged with, and knows something about, the world, rather than one who is simply 'sick' or malfunctioning. The 'strata' (stratification), we could say, are situated on the side of what is termed, following Lacan, the social Other of Demand and Language. In "How Do You Make Yourself a Body Without Organs?" (1987), Deleuze and Guattari situate the Body without Organs in opposition to the "organism", insist that "you have one, (or several)", and put forth an imperative for the subject to render, in an aesthetic act, the excess that constitutes the 'lost body' (without organs) into a productive subjective and social force. The authors champion particular social "practices", or modes of "experimentation", that produce the Body without Organs by rupturing the functionality of the organism.

> It's not so much that it [the Body without Organs] preexists or comes ready-made, although in certain respects it is preexistent ... you make one, you can't desire without making one. And it awaits you; it's an inevitable exercise or experimentation, already accomplished the moment you undertake it, unaccomplished the moment you don't. (p. 149)

It is interesting that, in this passage, the Body without Organs is linked to the question of desire—"you cannot desire without making one". It is well known that, on the question of desire, Deleuze and Guattari are ostensibly opposed to Lacan and psychoanalysis. For Deleuze and Guattari 'desire' is a purely productive force that bears no relation regarding its 'cause' to the negativity of Language and symbolic castration. For Lacan, however, the very existence and force of desire is founded upon a first inscription of lack (a traumatic loss) as a cause of desire itself. Deleuze and Guattari continue regarding the Body without Organs:

> This is not reassuring because you can botch it [Body without Organs]. Or it can be terrifying, and lead to your death. It is non-desire as well as desire. It is not at all a notion or a concept, but a practice, a set of practices. (pp. 149–150)

What is "non-desire"? And, what is it, as Deleuze and Guattari argue, that makes the psychotic's body fail as a "productive surface"? Must "non-desire" be situated at the point where the "experiment" fails, where the psychotic fails to create a Body without Organs, a resistant surface designed to create the conditions for a productive desire? Deleuze and Guattari's main charge here is that psychoanalysis "botches" the Body without Organs. "It [psychoanalysis] royally botches the real, because it botches the Body without Organs" (p. 151). Deleuze and Guattari claim that psychoanalysis botches the real/Body without Organs because psychoanalysis, in its approach, functions to 'Oedipalize' the psychotic.

> The error of psychoanalysis was to understand BwO phenomena as regressions, projections, phantasies, in terms of an image of the body. As a result, it only grasps the flipside of the Body without Organs and immediately substitutes family photos, childhood memories, and part objects for a worldwide intensity map. (p. 165)

Deleuze and Guattari set up a simple dichotomy consisting of the 'Oedipal' unified subject (organized and tyrannized within the family matrix and the State) versus the 'anti-oedipal' desiring 'multiplicity' whose force is not hemmed in by Oedipal familial or social structures. For Deleuze and Guattari, psychoanalysis is neuroticizing and repressive where "schizoanalysis" is schizophrenizing, and thus liberatory.

5.3 Conclusion: Towards an Ethics of the 'Body' of the Letter Beyond the Limits of the Law

Deleuze and Guattari's contention raises a serious question for psychoanalysis in the face of psychosis. Is the psychotic, left to psychoanalysis, in fact stranded, as Deleuze and Guattari argue, on the Oedipal plane? This last question will, in part, drive the inquiry regarding the problem of ethics in the following chapter. However, as a prelude, I will simply point to what potentially rescues psychoanalysis from functioning as one among many "technologies of the self"[2]: first, the status of the 'subject' insisted

[2] This is Michel Foucault's term for the deployment of disciplinary knowledge(s). See "Technologies of the Self" in *Technologies of the Self: A Seminar with Michel Foucault*, Ed. Luther, Martin, Hutton (1984).

upon in psychoanalysis and, second, the status of knowledge as it is revealed in the discourse of the psychotic. The 'subject' critiqued by Deleuze and Guattari, as for Foucault, is the Cartesian subject, which is also the object of critique for, it should be clear, Freud, Lacan, and psychoanalysis proper. As stated earlier, psychoanalysis confronts a subject of the unconscious that is defined by its very nature as the effect of the defect in signification and symbolic structure. The subject of psychoanalysis, as Lacan argued throughout, is not the Cartesian subject, but a subject (the subject as pure effect) of a radical exclusion caused by the cut of Language and the hole in knowledge.

As stated in the Introduction, I suggest that it is by following the ethic implicit in the knowledge (*savoir*) of the psychotic that psychoanalysis maintains its bearings as a praxis. However, to 'follow the psychotic' requires, as psychoanalyst Cantin (2002) writes, that "the analyst abandon any position that would refer to an ultimate Sense" (p. 95). Cantin's direction here presumes that both analyst and psychotic hold the same knowledge regarding the hole in knowledge, however from different positions in relation to the lost object and symbolic castration. So, regarding the question of the analyst's position vis-à-vis the knowledge (or truth) of the psychotic experience, we will stop here to underscore the necessity that the analyst's position be oriented towards a point beyond an Oedipal guarantee for "Sense" and meaning. Both the analyst and the psychotic, then, face the problem that arises from the lack of guarantee for Sense. For now, this last point will stand as a provisional response to Deleuze and Guattari's charge that the analyst is an agent of repression. To use Deleuze and Guattari's term, both analyst and the psychotic-becoming-analysand face the "Body without Organs" which holds the potential either for death or for the creation of life and difference.

It is in this sense that I raise the question of psychosis as, itself, the 'Body without Organs of psychoanalysis', i.e., the Body without Organs may operate as either a destructive or a productive limit for the psychotic—but for psychoanalysis as well. In other words, confronting psychosis with neurosis (an 'oedipalizing psychoanalysis') strands both the psychotic and psychoanalysis without recourse to what is at stake for the subject of the trauma. Deleuze and Guattari's conception of a "body without organs" is an echo of the conception of the 'body of the letter' outlined earlier following Freud and Lacan. Both phenomena (the body as 'letter' and "Body without Organs") locate resistant surfaces that function in the clinic as compass points to guide the analyst in the effort to contact under transference the subject of the unconscious of the psychotic.

References

Cantin, L. (2002). From delusion to dream. In R. Hughes & K. R. Malone (Eds.), *After Lacan: Clinical practice and the subject of the unconscious* (pp. 87–102). SUNY Press.

Deleuze, G., & Guattari, F. (1983). *Anti-Oedipus: Capitalism and Schizophrenia.* University of Minnesota Press.

Deleuze, G., & Guattari, F. (1987). How do you make yourself a body without organs? In *A thousand plateaus: capitalism and schizophrenia* (pp. 149–166). University of Minnesota Press.

Deleuze, G., & Parnet, C. (1987). *Dialogues* (H. Tomlinson, B. Habberjam, Trans.). Columbia University Press.

Deleuze, G. (1995). *Negotiations* (M. Joughin, Trans.). Columbia University Press.

Foucault, M. (1984). Technologies of the self. In L. Martin, H. Gutman, & P. Hutton (Eds.), *Technologies of the self: A seminar with Michel Foucault* (pp. 16–49). University of Massachusetts Press.

6

Towards a New Ethics

Ultimately, what I have to say here regarding ethics is in the service of the clinic of psychosis. In particular, my critique of ethics is from the perspective of the psychotic's discourse and my aim therefore is to improve our understanding of what is at stake in the psychoanalytic treatment of psychosis. I am dealing with one main question: What does the psychotic teach us about the Law?

Confronted with the psychotic's experience, we are compelled to examine the problem of ethics without recourse to the Good as installed and enforced by Oedipus. If we follow the psychotic, then we are faced with the failure of Oedipus at both the familial and social levels. I am not using the term ethics in the sense understood by North American practitioners in psychology or psychiatry as the code of professional ethics. Rather, I theorize the question of *ethics* by extracting the true stakes of Kant's moral Law (categorical imperative) by reading Kant after Lacan and in light of the psychotic's specific knowledge or *savoir*. The problem is that of constructing an *ethics without ethics*—in other words, an ethics without the guarantee of Aristotle's Good or Kant's "moral law within". Ultimately, this way of understanding ethics directly affects the clinic and

B. Fimiani, *Psychosis and Extreme States*, The Palgrave Lacan Series,
https://doi.org/10.1007/978-3-030-75440-2_6

potentially bears consequences for our conception of ethics in the social sphere as well.

In *Seminar III, The Psychoses*, Lacan (1993) theorized that the psychotic psychical structure is determined by a radical exclusion (*foreclosure*) of the primary word, or signifier, that, for neurotic subjects, comes to provide a first link in the subject's effort to make sense of experience. Thus the psychotic is without the primary, or fundamental, (symbolic) link to anchor the structure of psychical reality.

I argue that foreclosure is the result of the psychotic's first choice in life: a choice deployed at the moment of the *advent of the subject*. The psychotic's first choice is to radically exclude the symbolic anchoring point for Sense and meaning. Furthermore, I suggest that situating the psychotic's foreclosure as a choice is, in fact, the precondition for psychoanalysis and, by extension, the precondition for a new freedom for the psychotic subject. However, this first choice bears certain disastrous consequences for the subject of psychosis: without the anchoring point for Sense, she retreats into the closed universe of delusion and the 'violence' of the persecutory voices.

Yet it is of particular importance here to note that the psychotic's choice of foreclosure also yields a specific knowledge (*savoir*) regarding the foundation of the *Law* and the Ideals that support the rules of social coexistence. Simply put, the psychotic's *foreclosure* in turn exposes the Law, and the social rules that the Law supports, as unfounded. It is the psychotic's *savoir* of the Law that guides us in defining and theorizing an ethics and, furthermore, in formulating the aim of analysis as creating the conditions for a second (ethical) choice in the face of the effects of the Law that return when the delusion is ruptured. I argue that the psychotic's entrance into transference, defined as a desire-to-know, constitutes a second choice to enter the field of ethics and thus to assume a new responsibility for death drive. The psychotic, if given the place to speak, will reveal her subjective truth as well as the truth of the Law itself.

My thesis, then, is that there is a correspondence between the psychotic's *savoir* and the truth (or principle) behind the moral Law. The psychotic's *savoir* of the Law will take us further than even Lacan's powerful critique of Kantian ethics. The objective here is twofold: we aim to gain a clarified understanding of the moral Law itself, which, in turn, allows the analyst to better understand the symbolic (i.e., ethical) position required to invite the psychotic into the transference defined as a desire-to-know.

The psychotic will not respond, except with "indifference" (Freud's term) or paranoia, to anything other than the analyst's genuine desire 'to know' the truth of the psychotic's experience. Whereas Lacan based his interrogation of traditional ethics upon the neurotic's libidinal 'tie', we will allow the psychotic to lead the inquiry.

6.1 Clinical Stakes

In the clinic of psychosis, the term *ethics* ultimately regards (1) the action of the analyst in relation to the subject of the unconscious, and (2) the choice made by the psychotic analysand in light of the new knowledge produced in the course of the analytic experience. For both the analyst and the analysand the assumption of an ethical position always follows a certain experience under transference of the failure of symbolic and biological limits. So, what is the specific status of the said *act* and *choice* in the face of this failure of a universal limit?

I suggest that we must consider the field of ethics, and thus any true ethical act/choice, as a field produced in a moment of *rupture*, and in the moment of the subject's possible shift vis-à-vis the failure of a universal limit and thus the surging forth of an excess energy (or death drive). Furthermore, in the treatment of psychosis, the rupture is, simply put, that produced *in* delusion by the work of the dream and the simultaneous emergence of the subject. I will further elaborate the relation of dream to delusion. The aim of the psychoanalytic experience is the construction a new ethic for the subject. I deploy the term 'ethics' to capture and explain the subjective shift that may occur in the course of treatment wherein the subject of psychosis assumes a level of responsibility for her experience—hence my question regarding the function of 'choice' in the experience, and in the treatment of psychosis. The said 'shift' implies that the psychotic, in the course of treatment, moves from the position of an abused/persecuted 'object' to that of a speaking 'subject'.

Here I can return to the example,[1] referred to in Chap. 4, of a psychotic patient who, at a certain point in his treatment, raised a question about the 'truth' of his delusion. This patient termed a part of his delusion a "theory" and, at a particular moment, asked me: "Do you think there is any truth to it [to my theory]?" Until this moment in the treatment when the patient's question emerged, he spoke only with absolute certainty about being threatened with death by a persecutory Other that he called the "Circle of Supreme Beings". Prior to the emergence of his question the patient expressed no doubt regarding his delusion.

The emergence of the patient's question was significant (1) because the question emerged from *within* the patient (although provoked by the analyst) and (2) because the patient's question represents another path that is separate from the closed world of her delusion. With regard to this example, the key point, for now, is that with the emergence of the patient's question this person has a choice to make; she can either follow (elaborate) the question—as a path or opening out of delusion—or ignore the question regarding *truth* and cling to the certainty of her delusion.

The psychotic is surely faced with a choice here, as is any analysand who is in the throes of the analytic experience where she is confronted with the failure of the symptom and is therefore at a loss. The question for us is how does this choice differ for the psychotic versus the neurotic? As Lacan theorized, the neurotic has made a *forced choice* to enter Language and therefore has undergone a primary division as a subject. It is an open question as to whether or not the psychotic has ever made such a first choice, and the delusion—its characteristic certainty—suggests that she has not.

In order to explore the clinical relevance of this *choice* I will discuss the same clinical example further. There are three key moments in the treatment: (1) the emergence of the patient's delusion (a closed system), (2) the emergence of the dream which opposes delusion, and (3) a moment

[1] I noted in Chap. 4, although fictional, this clinical example is relevant in that it retains fundamental and generalizable truths of the psychotic experience and of the logic of treatment. In Chap. 4 the clinical example served to illustrate key points regarding the logic of dream-language versus the language of delusion. In the present chapter, key clinical moments are highlighted to explore how the *subject* of psychosis can challenge the certainty of delusional certainty.

near the end of the treatment when the patient questions the *truth* of her delusion.

6.2 Theoretical Stakes

The distinction between a first and second choice is key to maintaining the category of the psychotic's *savoir* as a *savoir* of the moral Law itself. In this chapter I will need to engage in a more extensive interrogation of the status of the Law and of *freedom* (i.e., choice) by way of Kant's *Critique of Practical Reason*, and in light of Lacan's reading of Kant in *Seminar VII* and in his 1963 essay "*Kant avec Sade*". I will return to Kant's notion of *respect* for the moral Law, and its relation to the principle behind the Law (a failed principle), to clarify this last point. In brief, *respect* for the Law alludes, paradoxically, to the *a priori* existence of the "moral law within", as Kant phrases it in his second *Critique*. What is the psychotic's relation (as subject) to Kant's notion of "respect" for the Law?

Furthermore, does Lacan go far enough in demonstrating that the Law, with its origin in the *faceless* voice as he puts it, is worse, more tyrannical, than even Kant theorized? The impetus for this last question is Gilles Deleuze and Felix Guattari's charge that psychoanalysis "botches the encounter with the psychotic", and ultimately with the Real (1983, 1987). The answer to the question raised by Deleuze and Guattari (does psychoanalysis botch the encounter with the psychotic?) depends upon the version of (perspective upon) the Law deployed by psychoanalysis in the treatment of psychosis. However, to achieve the said perspective upon the Law, psychoanalysis must choose to follow the psychotic's *savoir*. Following the psychotic, we witness a specific relation, and solution, to the faceless voice (an empty imperative).

In the face of the absence of a universal Good to guarantee one's choices in life, the subject is set adrift with only the question of desire (a lack-in-being) to guide the way. But this *lack* (desire) corresponds to the Law as both the cause and the object of the Law—that is, the Law as we know it after Kant's intervention in Aristotelian ethics.

6.3 Aristotle: The Function of the Good

With Aristotle the idea of the Good functioned as the foundation, and guide, in the pursuit of an ethics. In the *Nichomachean Ethics* (1975), Aristotle founds ethics by linking Happiness and pleasure to the Good; the Good as anchoring point, and as the *a priori* principle supporting ethics (the moral Law). Aristotle posited the Good as the guide to Happiness, and as the limit that ultimately defines and regulates *pleasure*. However, reading Aristotle, we must distinguish between the categories of "Pleasure" (as the Good itself) and "pleasure" as the (partial) satisfactions derived from one's effort to achieve the Good. Aristotle's definition of Pleasure as the Good itself is key.

In Book X of the *Ethics*, Aristotle suggests that "pleasure is the Good". We can grasp Aristotle's meaning (equating pleasure and the Good) via his comparison of pleasure with "motion" (p.280). Aristotle argues that the "true character of pleasure" is in fact the characteristic "completeness" of pleasure, such that pleasure is a "whole" (p. 281). Ultimately, Aristotle's comparison between pleasure and motion regards a distinction between that which occurs "in time" versus that which occurs in a "moment". The "moment" is self-contained (whole) whereas that which occurs "in time" is subject to certain divisions. Aristotle elaborates this distinction and he begins, interestingly, with the phenomenon of ("complete") "vision":

> We regard an act of vision as complete at any given moment: it *lacks nothing* which has to develop later in order to make complete the specific form that constitutes the act of seeing. Something similar seems to be true of pleasure also: it is a whole, and one cannot at a given moment find a pleasure whose specific form will be brought to completion only if the pleasure lasts longer. That is precisely why pleasure is not motion. For all motion—take building, for example—takes place in time and is directed at an end; it is complete only when it has accomplished that at which it aims. (italics added, p. 280)

What emerges here is a clear sense, in Aristotle, that Pleasure, and thus the Good, exists in a full state outside of time and its imperatives. Aristotle continues, further situating pleasure on the side of a certain (desirable) fullness or "whole":

> But pleasure completes the activities, and consequently life, which they ["men"] desire. No wonder, then, that men also aim at pleasure: each man finds that it *completes his life*, and his life is desireable. (italics added, p. 282)

The Pleasure that "completes his life", I suggest, differs from the multiple 'pleasures' that Aristotle describes as possible for the human. The Good is "whole", yet a wholeness that is, even according to Aristotle, missing from one's life, thus, as Aristotle puts it, rendering the Good "desireable", and leaving one's life (experience) "full" of desire, that is, one's experience is full of a *lack of the Good.* What is situated as the Good is a "whole" or "complete" Pleasure, yet a Pleasure that when achieved *completes one's life.*

Viewed through a Freudian lens, Pleasure (that which "completes his life") is situated on the side of death, and of *total satisfaction.* The status of Pleasure leads to an economic imperative: the Good represents a certain excess (Enjoyment) that, because it is lacking, regulates pleasure(s) in life. Moreover, Aristotle polices the division between 'desire' and Pleasure (excess) with moral prescriptions designed to bar access to a subjective state of *too much* or *too little*; Aristotle's suggested middle path, as Lacan says in *Seminar VII* (1992), constitutes a "cleaning up of desire" characteristic of "traditional ethics" (p. 314).

The key point here is that, although unattainable, the Good (for Aristotle) is nonetheless 'Good-in-itself'. In other words, the Good maintains a certain positive 'value' and therefore represents a 'wholeness' that is both worth waiting for (desiring) and consequently worth dying for, i.e., Pleasure (the Real) is possible, however 'you must wait'! According to Aristotle, the Good, as an *a priori* principle, is infinite and thus founds ethics and the moral Law itself.

With the requirement of the Good to found ethics, we arrive at what constitutes, as Alenka Zupancic (2000) argues in "Ethics of the Real", the "fundamental paradox of ethics". As Zupancic observes, "in order to found an ethics, we already have to presuppose a certain ethics (a certain notion of the good)" (p. 92).

Kant confronts this paradox, an impasse, with the categorical imperative.

6.4 Kant: The "Moral Law Within"

Juliet Flower MacCannell (2000) writes of the shift in the status of the Good that occurred in the eighteenth century which precipitated a certain 'crisis' in traditional ethics. Here MacCannell underscores the historico-libidinal context for the crisis in ethics:

> After Kant and Rousseau, no one was permitted to count their own good in any ethical process. Nor their own "goodness" either, as the very quality of goodness was contaminated by the aggressive drive from which it originally stemmed. (pp. 67–68)

The removal of the Good from both individual and sociopolitical considerations bore certain consequences in the field of ethics and "morality". MacCannell continues: "Thus, with these two thinkers, the Good was disqualified as the determinant of individual and social reason, respectively" (p. 68). We must keep both the 'individual' and 'social' registers in mind because the psychotic's singular (individual) *savoir* pertains to the defect in the social fabric, the social link. The analyst must know this fact intimately or risk meeting the psychotic with Oedipal requirements which are tied to an illusion of the Good, and for which the psychotic has no use.

With Kant we witness an attempt to found an ethics, not with reference to an *a priori* Good, as in Aristotle, but with a concept of the Law as founded in 'itself'. For Kant, the Good (posited as universal) is inseparable from the "pathological" or libidinal ties of the individual subject. The Good, then, is rendered problematic because the Good, Kant concluded, is derived from "pathological" incentives or 'drives' that inevitably *contaminate* the supposed ethical act itself. The result in Kant's moral philosophy (of the overturning of the Good) was the "categorical imperative" which states: "Act so that the maxim of your will can hold at the same time as the principle giving universal law."

On its face the categorical imperative appears designed to rid ethics of the "pathological", thus creating the possibility of a *pure* ethics. We must observe, however, that Kant's solution leaves us with a more difficult problem or *paradox*, namely the fact that there is no way to determine if one's will (the "maxim of your will") corresponds to the "principle giving [supporting] universal law". Yes, Kant gives the 'choice' (decision) to the individual, yet leaves open the question of what precisely qualifies as the criterion for universality in the individual's calculation of his or her "act".[2] Of course, that which is 'universal' is supposed by Kant to be what is *good* for all. Thus to act in conformity with Kant's categorical imperative one must know the *good* at the moment of, or before, one's act.

Is the paradox produced by Kant's categorical imperative of a different sort than that produced by Aristotelian ethics? Both the Aristotelian and Kantian approaches to ethics, despite Kant's sweeping away of the Good as such, end up with the problem of the cause, or origin, of the moral Law. More precisely, both Aristotle and Kant produce the said paradox in the attempt to establish the origin and status of the individual's attachment, or libidinal investment, to/in the Law as imperative to serve the 'Good' or the 'universal' respectively.

Kant attempts to answer the question of the individual's investment in the Law by positing the existence of the "moral Law within". We can hear Kant's personal revelation regarding the origin, and internal effect, of the Law in the Conclusion to his second *Critique* (1956): "Two things fill the mind with ever new and increasing admiration and awe ... the starry heavens above me and the moral law within me" (p. 166). Kant continues, and here we might note the way in which he situates the "law within" as coextensive with the advent of the "self":

> The latter ["law within"] begins at my invisible self, my personality, and exhibits me in a world which has true infinity but which is comprehensible only to the understanding—a world in which I recognize myself as existing in a universal and necessary ... connection, and thereby also in connection with all those visible worlds. (p. 166)

[2] See Alenka Zupancic's *Ethics of the Real* (2000) for an elaboration of this second paradox that is implicit in Kant's categorical imperative and its relation to the question of the correspondence between an 'ethical act' and the categories of "Good and Evil" (pp. 92–105).

The Law is the means through which the "invisible self" comes to be anchored (finds "connection" and "existence") in the face of "true infinity," and in the face of an "unbounded magnitude of worlds beyond worlds and systems beyond systems" (p. 166). As Kant says, "the former view (a "boundless magnitude") annihilates ... my importance as an animal creature" (p. 166). Against this "annihilation" of the individual by the "multitude" Kant responds with the "law" to give "worth" to the individual. The "moral law within",

> on the contrary, infinitely raises my worth as that of an intelligence by my personality, in which the moral law reveals a life independent of all animality and even of the whole world of sense—*at least so far as it may be inferred from the purposive destination assigned to my existence by this law.* (italics added, p. 166)

But, for the psychotic, the question is: What is so compelling about Kant's experience of assignation such that his *existence in* the Law, or of the Law *in* him, is made possible?

6.5 The "Precondition for the Worth of the Person": "Pain" versus "Respect"

In the chapter of his second *Critique* entitled "The Incentives of Pure Practical Reason", Kant argues that the only non-pathological "incentive" or "feeling" that may guide the individual's acceptance of the Law is what he terms "respect" for the moral Law. But this formulation ('acceptance of the Law') is problematic in itself because, as we have already discussed, it is the "paradox" of ethics (the requirement for an *a priori* support for the Law) that Kant attempts to solve.

When he defines "respect" Kant reveals the true difficulty presented by the paradox. On the one hand, Kant writes: "Respect for the moral law ... is the only one [moral 'feeling'] which we can know completely a priori" (p. 76). Yet, in a subsequent passage Kant indicates that "respect", the emergence of the feeling of respect in the subject, coincides, or perhaps is, the Law itself. Kant argues:

> In the subject there is no antecedent feeling tending to morality; that is impossible, because all feeling is sensuous, and the incentives of the moral disposition must be free from every sensuous condition. (p. 78)

What Kant suggests is that, by contrast, "sensuous feeling … is the condition of the moral feeling we call respect" (p. 78). Thus, he concludes, "because of its origin", respect can only be said to be "practically", not "pathologically", effected; in other words, respect is a "moral feeling", as Kant writes, "produced solely by reason" (p. 78).

> Thus respect for the law is not the incentive to morality; *it is morality itself, regarded subjectively as an incentive*, inasmuch as pure practical reason, [that] by rejecting all the rival claims of self-love, gives authority and absolute sovereignty to the law. (italics added, pp. 78–79)

The key to understanding what is at stake in Kant's conclusion is the phrase "regarded subjectively as an incentive". Something happens *in* the individual, Kant suggests, that renders the effect of the Law as the *individual's* "incentive" (his or her *own* "moral feeling") versus an external and thus pure imperative or invasive command.

So, for Kant there is an *effect* in the individual that in turn produces respect as a moral feeling. As Kant says, his aim is to show what the Law "effects (or better, must effect) in the mind, so far as it is an incentive" (p. 75). "It" (ostensibly the Law) is an "incentive", yet only insofar as the feeling or incentive of "respect" is produced in the individual. And, furthermore, "respect" is "morality itself".

What is hidden here where the *production* of the Law and the individual's "respect" for the Law occur simultaneously?

In his explanation of the relation of "respect" to "humiliation", Kant himself provides a guide to illuminating the hidden aspect of the individual's experience. Kant explains that respect and humiliation correspond to two separate possibilities in the event of the confrontation between the Law, on one side, and "self-conceit" on the other. He opens the question (regarding the "determination of the will through the moral law") via the juxtaposition of the "negative" versus the "positive" effects of the Law. Kant describes the purely "negative effect of the law" and its result—"pain":

> Thus far, the effect of the moral law as an incentive is only negative, and as such can be known a priori. For all inclination and every sensuous impulse is based on feeling, and the negative effect on feeling (through the check on the inclinations) is itself feeling. Consequently, we can see a priori that the moral law as a ground of determination of the will, by thwarting all our inclinations, must produce a feeling which can be called pain. (p. 75)

In this passage, we get the sense that the law is demanding 'too much' of the individual, hence the "pain". The "negative effect" of the law acts as a "check" on "inclination" and "sensuous impulse". But Kant is pursuing the question of how, by what means, the movement from the purely "negative" to the "positive" effect of the law occurs. The negative effect appears to mark a subjective experience of the law that is, by definition, prior to the emergence of "respect".

What is at stake in the movement, in the individual, from the negative to the positive effect of the law? Kant writes:

> All inclinations taken together (which can be brought into a fairly tolerable system, whereupon their satisfaction is called happiness) constitute self-regard (*solipsismus*). (p. 76)

Kant divides "self-regard" into "self-love" and "self-conceit". Whereas "self-love" is merely "checked" (limited) by the law, and thus allowed to persist as "rational self-love", "self-conceit", by contrast, is 'struck' down (p. 76). The "strike" by the law to "self-conceit" is what produces "humiliation" versus "happiness". The aim of the law in striking down self-conceit, ultimately, is to bring the will into "agreement" with the law (p. 76). This "agreement", as Kant says, is the "first condition of any worth of the person" (p. 76).

As we know, following Lacan, this "agreement" is impossible for any subject of Language. Furthermore, the psychotic presents a specific challenge to this requirement to be in 'agreement' with the Law. It is unclear whether Kant requires a *total* agreement with the Law, but I would suggest that the psychotic does not enter into this problematic of agreement at all; neither total agreement nor any form of agreement which implies some compromise vis-à-vis loss (e.g., the "check on the inclinations"). Kant continues that "any presumption [of worth] prior to this ['strike'] is false and opposed to the law" (p. 76). What Kant terms the "self-conceit" (or "arrogance") of the individual, I call the *savoir* of the unconscious: a *savoir* that Kant attempts to cover over, to keep *hidden.*

In the moment of the "strike" to self-conceit (a negation of "happiness/satisfaction"), and the subsequent "humiliation" and "pain", does the individual have the *choice* of "respect" versus some other response, for example, terror? Or, does "respect" somehow take the place of what would otherwise be pure terror given a failure of the moral law to confer "worth?" We will develop this point further following Lacan, but first let us follow Kant further on this question. Kant writes that "as striking down, i.e., humiliating, self-conceit, it [the law] is an object of the greatest respect" (p. 76).

> Since the idea of the moral law deprives self-love of its influence and self-conceit of its delusion, it lessens the obstacle to pure practical reason and produces the idea of the superiority of its objective law to the impulses of sensibility. (p. 78)

It is here that Kant concludes that respect is "morality itself", not merely an "incentive" *to* morality. Something is repressed here, in Kant, that separates terror from humiliation and, subsequently, pain from respect.

In fact, Kant does not characterize "respect" as a choice per se, but as, again, something that acts (mysteriously) in the individual and that functions to (simultaneously) designate the moral law as such, i.e., to give the law worth and "absolute sovereignty" (p. 79). The mysterious force of "respect" for the law is most evident in an example that Kant himself provides. Kant's objective in the following example is to maintain a strict distinction between respect and *inclinations* such as fear, love, admiration, and awe. For example, where fear may be present regarding a particular other (man or woman), Kant says that "inner respect for him may still be lacking" (p. 79). Quoting the eighteenth-century French philosopher Fontanelle, Kant writes: "I bow to a great man, but my mind does not bow." Kant continues with his own commentary:

> I can add [to Fontanelle]: to a humble plain man, in whom I perceive righteousness in a higher degree than I am conscious of in myself, *my mind bows* whether I choose to or not. … Why? His example holds a law before me which strikes down my self-conceit when I compare my own conduct with it; that it is a law that can be obeyed, and consequently is one that can be put into practice, is proved to my eyes by the act. (author's italics, pp. 79–80)

There are two points we can draw from this last quote: (1) that Kant's qualifying phrase "whether I choose to or not" implies a more fundamental choice that has, subsequently, rendered the mind's "bow" obligatory, and (2) while it is clear that the "worth" of the individual is contingent upon respect (versus "self-conceit"), it is the "worth" of the Law itself that is conferred by the bow (the sign of "inner respect"), that is, as Kant writes, following the individual's bow "it is a law that can be obeyed" (p. 80). In other words, that which mysteriously acts in the individual—that which responds with "respect" to "pain" in the proper way—*simultaneously* brings the subject and the Law into existence. For Kant it is "inner respect" which functions as the "sole and undoubted moral incentive" that determines the will and thus establishes the worth of the moral law itself.

Is it not the psychotic who demonstrates a "presumption of worth", but without reference to the Law, thus rendering the lack in the law (as both castration and cause of desire) ineffectual in the psychotic's universe? Here we must separate the true *lack* in the Law (the Other) from the psychotic solution deployed to repress or fill the lack, that is, delusion.

6.5.1 The Delusion Is Lawless

We can rely upon the patient I have introduced earlier to explore and provide clinical ground for this last question. With the foreclosure of the Name-of-the-Father, and therefore the Law, the psychotic subject retreats into a closed universe of delusion, a universe where the subject is reduced to an object of aggression. In the initial phase of his treatment this patient elaborated a delusion in which he was a victim.

In the early phase of the treatment the patient's discourse consisted of pure delusion. The structure of the delusion emerged during the first phase of treatment, and its stability rested upon the functioning of four elements. The main elements include the opposition between two forces—the "evil and kind voices"—which are controlled by a third authoritarian and omnipotent force represented by the "Circle of Supreme Beings". The "evil voices" constantly berate him and threaten to "kill his mother and brother" if, for example, he "talks back" to the voice, that is, the patient (or their mother/brother) will be killed if he does "what he wants". In other words, for him, to desire = death in the scheme of his delusion; he will "be killed".

In addition to occupying the position of an abused object or victim, this patient's delusion also afforded him a contrary position of a *chosen one*, or agent, who could achieve great things. He spoke of being required by the "Supreme Beings" to be a "Nobel Laureate". Although this requirement is impossible for the patient to achieve, there appears to be a "presumption of worth" conferred upon him given that he is able to manufacture a potentially vital role for himself—the role of a Nobel Laureate, however impossible that may be.

So, the fourth element of his delusion regards his position in the face of the impossible demand of the "Supreme Beings". He is positioned between the "evil" and "kind" voices, whom the "Supreme Beings" control. The patient describes that his only recourse is to wait for the "Supreme Beings" to intervene and stop the voices—which, the patient told me, they never do. His delusion is a closed system that leaves him at an impasse. By impasse I mean that there is no space for the subject, for any lack, in the scheme of his delusion. Even with the demand/requirement to be a Nobel Laureate, the patient is relegated to the position of a passive object.

As I mentioned earlier, later in the treatment this same patient raises a question about the "truth" of his delusion. However, in the beginning phase of the treatment, described here, his delusion remained totalizing, without lack. Figure 6.1 provides the structure of his delusion.

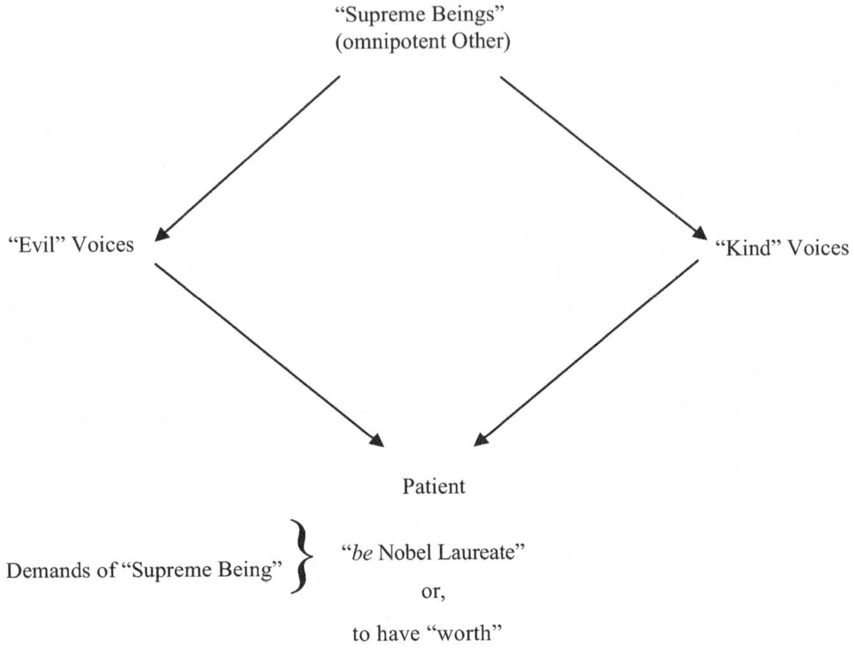

Fig. 6.1 Structure of delusion

This vignette helps us understand how the psychotic obtains some sense of "worth" outside the Law. The totalizing quality of the delusion is the hallmark of the psychotic's discourse and is also the sign that the Law is not functioning in the psychical life of the psychotic. The delusion 'confers worth on the person' but without any submission to, and functioning of, the Law.

Where the Law is radically excluded—where there is no limit or protection typically supplied by the Law—the Other is left non-barred. In Fig. 6.1, the "Supreme Beings" occupy the place of a non-barred/non-castrated Other. As this patient once said, "the Supreme Beings control the voices … no one controls the Supreme Beings". The "Supreme Beings" are not subjected to the Law—they are the Law itself. The delusion is born of the psychotic subject's specific knowledge of the failure of the Law to protect. Furthermore, in treatment, under transference, the patient may face the possibility of losing the delusion. For example, my patient's "question" ('Do you think there is any truth to it [to my theory]?') marks the onset of this loss for my patient. However, what will the psychotic follow, if not the delusion that maintains the illusion of wholeness? The difficulty for the psychotic is to lose the 'presumption of worth *without* the Law' (which is manifest in the grandiosity of delusion) and face the essential "worthlessness" of, or *lack in*, the Law. When I say the 'lack in the Law' I imply something Other to the Law—something that is in the Law but that is nonetheless not lawful.

As I will explore further, the subject's (any subject's) primary response to the *voice* in the Law is *terror*. However, whereas the neurotic deploys respect (or repression) to find protection from the command of the voice, the psychotic by contrast moves from terror to certainty and the protection afforded by the delusion.

6.6 Lacan: The Thing and the Obscene "Voice" (of the Law)

What is the cost for the subject in the "agreement" between the will and the moral law? Kant is silent on this point. Thus we will turn to Lacan to give a voice to what is at stake where the subject is forced to choose between annihilation and the double effect of the Law. Fundamental to Lacan's perspective is that the moral voice "within" must be resisted by the subject. In *Seminar VII*, regarding the patient's "moral experience", Lacan asks:

> Will it or will it not submit itself to the duty that it feels within like a stranger ... should it or should it not submit itself to the half-conscious, paradoxical, and morbid command of the superego. ... If I may put it thus, *isn't its true duty to oppose that command*? (italics mine, p. 7)

First we must note that the "it" in question in Lacan's statement ("will it submit...") is the subject itself. Thus "its true duty to oppose that command" regards "it" as the subject of, and in, the Law. Second, the true stakes of ethics in psychosis must be set beyond the form of the initial question framed by Lacan in the quote. For example, as Lacan goes on to say, the (moral) question "should it, or should it not…" is typical of the obsessional neurotic's quest at the beginning of the analysis. I suggest that the field of ethics opens precisely at the point where the subject faces a void that is beyond the question of the "worth" of the imperative, or Law.

Furthermore, it is not clear that we can apply Lacan's dictum—to resist, in particular, the superegoic command—directly to psychosis given that the psychotic is always beyond the question of whether to resist the superego "or not", i.e., the question of 'compromise', of being divided in the face of the Law, is *foreclosed* for the psychotic. The psychotic makes a first choice to foreclose the effect of loss, thus installing an absolute and omnipotent Other typical of delusion. Nonetheless, if we modify Lacan's position regarding the 'command' just slightly, he does provide a guide to an ethical position, for example, when Lacan suggests that "its [the subject's] true duty is to oppose [contest] that command". In order to include the psychotic's particular dilemma in the face of the Law, we might say that both analysand and analyst have a *duty* to the subject in order to *oppose* the commands of the superego (neurosis) *and delusional certainty* (psychosis). Thus we have an initial sense of an *ethics* (a new responsibility) that becomes necessary in a field that is beyond neurotic Ideals and psychotic certainty—beyond any command.

6.6.1 A Forced Choice: Terror or "Respect"

Now we can confront directly, with a Lacanian logic, the choice that is merely implied in the previous quote by Kant (to bow "whether I choose to or not"). In *Seminar XI* (1978), on the subject's fundamental alienation, Lacan deploys the choice "your money or your life" to capture the nature of the subject's primary confrontation with the Law, and with the first imperative to 'choose' between "being" and "meaning", a 'forced choice'. In neurosis, the forced choice results in a compromise—you get your life (meaning) but without your money (being/enjoyment)—thus producing a *subject of neurosis* and *lack*. To use the Kantian term, we could say that the neurotic deploys "respect" to justify (repress) the true cost of this first (forced) choice. I suggest that the neurotic's choice—or more aptly the choice of neurosis—creates a path for the subject towards the dialectic of desire (and love/seduction), thus avoiding a direct confrontation with a pure *terror* in the face of annihilation.

Does "respect" require the 'existence' (representation) of primary repression? And thus, does respect for the law, specifically in psychosis, give way to terror as the prevailing (i.e., conscious) experience of the Law and its requirement of loss? To begin, I suggest that the psychotic, without recourse to the Name-of-the-Father, and in the face of radical terror, makes a (first) choice that allows no compromise and thus requires a totalizing knowledge as a solution to the terror. I contend that the psychotic's first choice (and its solution) makes a *second choice* (under transference) doubly difficult because the second choice is perceived as pure "evil" (as radically outside) and thus constitutes a true ethical choice.[3]

In her study of ethics, Zupancic (2000) is instructive on the presence of the "terror" that is inherent in the forced choice:

> The ultimate act of terror, the most radical terror, is when we are forced to subjectivize ourselves, when we are forced to choose—we must do so, and thus demonstrate that we are free subjects, whether we want to or not. (p. 213)

Zupancic's formulation of the contingency of radical terror and freedom runs parallel to Kant's formulation on the action of "respect" in the individual—yet with one crucial difference. Following Lacan, Zupancic identifies "terror" (a terror at the core of the subject) that is fundamental to the subject's investment in, and thus support for, the "worth" of the Law.

It is *terror* (the truth of the subject) that is repressed in Kant's version, not simply of the Law, but of the individual's (libidinal) investment in the Law. From a Lacanian perspective, the truth of the subject corresponds to (is) the truth of/in the Law. "Respect", which is Kant's version of the truth of/in the law, represses the (w)hole in the law and its corresponding terror. In contrast, Lacan is interested in the subject's knowledge or *savoir* of a particular terror in the face of the forced choice presented by the Law.

[3] I will later define the ethical act as "evil" insofar as the act is perceived as such from the point of view of certainty, insofar as certainty is the antithesis of the effect of a rupture or event. The question of "terror" also recalls the Deleuzian conception of the Body without Organs as the frontier of either terror (death) or desire (life).

6.7 Psychosis: The Hole in the Law, and the Return of an Excess in the 'voice'

What is the mysterious object in the Law that, for Kant, evokes "respect" in place of "pain/humiliation", yet, from a Lacanian perspective, provides a distinction between terror and respect? And why does the psychotic respond to the *object* in the Law with terror? To approach these questions I begin with the following Lacanian premise: The 'terror' evoked by the Law stems from the effect (in the subject) of the lost *object* in the Law: *das Ding*. The Thing, we will see, is an experience in the body of the potential violence of the Law and its return in the body as an internal object: the voice.

After Kant the Law becomes a moral *voice* that speaks from within—a voice that strikes fear into the individual. In his second *Critique* Kant writes: "as practical reason presents it [moral law] to us for obedience, whose voice makes even the boldest sinner tremble and forces him to hide himself from it" (p. 82). More importantly, following Lacan, Kant's Law (as voice) becomes an (internal) object which the individual can then *hear* as though "broadcast" from a point in space. Lacan (2006) writes in "Kant with Sade":

> Let us observe that the herald of the maxim need be no more here than a point of broadcast. It could be a voice on the radio. ... Such voice-related phenomena, especially those found in psychosis, truly have this object-like appearance. And in its early days, psychoanalysis was not very far from relating the voice of conscience to psychosis. (p. 650)

How does Lacan arrive at such a thesis which states that the voice of the Law (the moral imperative) is "object-like" and, more importantly, that the object (voice) is something like that found in the phenomenology of psychosis? For the subject the 'voice of the law' is not a strictly benevolent force. Rather, the voice of the law is a force that, by definition, betrays our very 'being' in favour of Sense.

In "Kant with Sade", Lacan draws the force for his argument by demonstrating the way in which Sade's maxim (to enjoy) reveals the hidden truth of Kant's moral imperative. Lacan relates Sade's maxim in the following way:

> "I have the right to enjoy your body," anyone can say to me, "and I will exercise this right without any limit to the capriciousness of the exactions I may wish to satiate with your body." (p. 648)

The point here is embodied in the phrase "anyone can say to me", which right away locates the origin of the maxim in the Other, that is, "anyone [the other/Other] can say to me" that it is my "right" to enjoy/abuse you/me; I have absolute power over you/me—but it is "I" who gives the Other such power. At the level of the statement, the paradox in Sade's maxim is that the subject ("I") speaks as though it is the origin and author of what it says. As Lacan writes,

> [i]n coming out of the Other's mouth, Sade's maxim is more honest than Kant's appeal to the voice within, since it unmasks the split in the subject that is usually covered up. (p. 650)

By including the "anyone can say to me", Sade reveals the truth of the subject (of enunciation/unconscious) as fundamentally alienated in its confrontation with the Law. Lacan's reading of Sade reveals the fact that,

> [...] the bipolarity upon which the moral law is founded is nothing but the split in the subject brought about by any and every intervention of the signifier [...] (p. 650)

Sade's maxim offers a *rule* for the exchange of *jouissance*, yet it is a rule accompanied by the command to enjoy/abuse the other and be enjoyed/abused by the Other as its basic *principle*. So we can hold the principle behind Sade's and (after Lacan) Kant's imperative in contrast to that of Aristotle. Where Aristotle's Supreme Good (as principle) functions to delimit the "middle path", thus limiting excess (*jouissance*), Kant (with Sade) posits a Law whose principle fails to regulate the pleasure–pain continuum. Moreover, as Lacan writes in *Seminar VII*, at the core of the moral law is the imperative (characteristic of the Freudian "super-ego") to achieve (possess) the impossible, e.g., to obtain the irrevocably lost object, the "Thing".

In the chapter entitled "On the Moral Law" in *Seminar VII*, Lacan says:

> On the horizon, beyond the pleasure principle, there rises up the *Gut, das Ding*, thus introducing at the level of the unconscious something that ought to oblige us to ask once again the Kantian question of the *causa noumenon*. (p. 73)

The *Gut*, the Good, is equated, after Lacan's intervention, with *das Ding*, or the Thing, which inevitably corresponds to the subject and which in turn leads the subject (ultimately) to its satisfaction and death, i.e., the Thing is, ultimately, *too good*. Lacan says: "[H]e [the subject] cannot stand the extreme good that *das Ding* may bring him" (p. 73). So the command of the moral imperative necessarily becomes: you must do '*x*' which may bring you 'good' (take you to an extreme)—and there is no guarantee, neither biological nor symbolic, to stop the subject from going too far, e.g., from having it *too good* (or, for the psychotic, of making it too good for the Other).

Lacan illuminates the stakes for the subject in the face of the lack of any guarantee, and in the face of the void opened up by the lack in the Law:

> *Das Ding* presents itself at the level of unconscious experience as that which already makes the law. Although it is necessary to give this verbal phrase, "makes the law," the emphasis it receives in one of the most brutal games of elementary society. … It is a capricious and arbitrary law, the law of the oracle, the law of signs in which the subject receives no guarantee from anywhere. (p. 73)

This is the law as pure *voice*, and as "brutal" in the sense that it provides the subject with no ultimate Sense for loss, and with which she might guard herself against the truth of loss. Lacan continues, further elaborating the capricious aspect of the law with no "guarantee from anywhere", indicating "the law in which he [the subject] receives no *Sicherung*, to use another Kantian term" (p. 73). The German *Sicherung* translates to

English as both *safety* (*Sich* = safe) and *security/securing*, but also as *protection*—as in 'the subject receives protection from the brutality of the law'.

It is precisely the psychotic's experience of an initial trauma, instituted by Language, that corresponds to what Lacan describes as the "brutal games of elementary society", for example, where the 'first' loss occurs that is contingent upon the eruption of the voice—an eruption prior to the *existence* of the signifier as such. Most important is that, unlike the neurotic, the psychotic does not pass to another subject position in which she would obtain the protection (*Sicherung*) of the signifier, and of Sense—protection, thus, against the return of the Thing (in the voice) and of the return of the object that falls from the voice (in the body).

6.7.1 The Question(ing) of the Universal

Kant's proposal of "respect" as the mechanism designed to situate the moral law "within" does so at the cost of the subject itself and the utility of the Thing as a guide to an ethics. More specifically, and regarding the stakes for the psychotic, the path to "respect" for the law, I suggest, is a path marked by the signifier, and thus a path *chosen* by the neurotic who, by definition, bears the protection offered by the signifier and of the universal as such. Such an ethics, reliant upon an *a priori* universal, is not credible or of much use to the subject of the psychotic experience. However, this does not preclude the possibility that, under transference, the psychotic may successfully confront, and come to terms with, the question of the universal. The question of the universal of course implies the Law's inherent lack or failure to protect.

Given the failure of the subject to confer *worth* upon the Law (and vice versa), the psychotic moves from terror to certainty, and thus moves from the *possibility* of becoming a desiring (split) subject to a pure object of/for the Other's enjoyment. The result of the first choice (the direct passage from terror to certainty) is that the psychotic is without any choice (freedom) whatsoever. In the schema of my patient's delusion (Fig. 6.1) we can see that he is left in a position without freedom. Our concern is that of creating a new possibility for a second choice.

6.8 From the Absence of a Good to the Requirement of a New Ethic Through Transference

Thus we move towards the question of a *second* choice that, I argue, may occur under the constraints of transference defined as a desire-to-know—a desire for *savoir* (knowledge) coming from the unconscious. First, I will define and explore the status of the ethical act itself, and then I will examine what the implications are for such an act regarding the positions of the analyst and the psychotic in treatment.

The ethical act itself requires the emergence of something new: for instance, the emergence of a potential for the reconfiguration of what *exists* (structurally). With regard to the structure of psychosis, I define the status of the "something new" as the emergence of *lack* itself.

The formal (structural) difference between delusion and dream, and their juxtaposition in the speech of the patient create the conditions for contestation, and thus for a *rupture* as pure potentiality. Following psychoanalysts Apollon et al. (2002), we must begin with the premise that the delusion has a specific function, and that, to begin the treatment, the analyst must take what the psychotic says (his delusion) literally insofar as the delusion functions as a theory of a *truth* that the psychotic knows. The dream functions to pierce a hole in the delusion, thus creating the possibility for the psychotic to reverse her position and question the certainty of delusion. However, the said possibility for a new position for the subject, I suggest, hinges upon the production of an ethic in the face of the rupture introduced by the dream; this last point opens the way to a full exploration of *ethics*.

Finally, it is the said reversal of the psychotic's position, vis-à-vis delusional certainty, that marks the 'installation' of transference defined as a desire-to-know. I am here defining transference as a desire for knowledge coming from the unconscious. This is a knowledge that, if properly supported by the analyst, will contest the certainty of delusion. In the case I am discussing, the dream functions as the gateway to his unconscious.

6.8.1 The Emergence of the Dream

Returning to the clinical example, once the patient had elaborated his delusion, represented in Fig. 6.1, I asked him to try to remember his dreams and to speak about his dreams in session. Following my intervention he reported the following dream which he stated was "about his dad": "*He was driving with me in the car, I guess that's when I was a younger man, and I thought he was asleep and I woke up and tried to catch the steering wheel, before we have a wreck.*" In session he further elaborated that in the dream he feared that "they would die" because the father was "asleep at the wheel". In the dream, however, he was able to "grab the wheel" and avert the crash. This dream also led the patient to elaborate new material from his personal history including childhood memories with his father. Most importantly, this dream recalled a childhood memory, much like the dream scene but with a critical difference, where the patient was in the car with his father and his father was falling asleep. However, his position in the memory was quite different from his position in the dream in that, in the memory, the patient was unable to move or to wake his father. In other words, in the memory the patient sat passively and in fear of "crashing" and of "being killed".

At stake here is the fact that his dream emerged in response to the desire of the analyst and that the dream evoked the first material in the treatment that is outside of delusion. Furthermore, the dream introduced new material from his personal history that underscored his subjective position (in fear of death) and in the presence of his father's seemingly 'negligent' act of being "asleep at the wheel". In retrospect I now situate the emergence of this dream and its associations as a force in opposition to the closed world of his delusion. We could say that with the emergence of his dream, and memory, his unconscious has 'acted' and produced new material. And I suggest that this act of the unconscious is in opposition to the aim of his delusion. The dream produces an opening whereas the aim of the delusion is to form a whole. The following provides a juxtaposition of the elements of delusion versus the new elements evoked by the dream:

Delusion	Dream/Memories
"Supreme Beings"	Patient's "father"
"You must..."	"father falling asleep"
"you will be killed"	father "killing [us]"
	"I can't do anything"

Yet we must insist upon a distinction here; the ethical act itself is constituted by more than the simple emergence of an opposition and potential rupture. What is required on the patient's side is a 'choice' that affirms the rupture as such, i.e., the rupture is pure potential that represents the possibility for a reconfiguration of the subject's relation to death drive, and thus another way to be in the world. Again the question is: 'will the patient choose to follow the dream, or remain committed to the familiar territory of delusion?

The relation of the first (forced) choice to a 'second' choice under transference is fundamental to the operation of psychoanalysis in general. Zupancic (2000), in her synthesis of Lacan and Kant, makes this relation clear when she writes the following:

> The claim that the subject ... chooses her unconscious—which might be called the psychoanalytic postulate of freedom—is the very condition of possibility of psychoanalysis. The change of perspective that occurs at the end of analysis ... can only occur against the background of this postulate. This initial choice can be repeated—the analysis comes to its conclusion as it brings the subject to the threshold of another (a second) choice, *that is, when the subject finds once again the possibility of choice.* (italics added, p. 35)

In confronting psychosis, the "postulate of freedom" as the precondition for psychoanalysis, generally holds. For the purpose of our argument, we might add that the postulate of freedom is the precondition of a practice of psychoanalysis in which the question of ethics is the guide. Furthermore, while the *end of analysis* is relevant, here we are discussing the *installation* of transference and thus the beginning of treatment. And the particular subject in question is the subject of psychosis whose experience of the return of this *initial* choice necessarily differs. The psychotic's relation to the forced choice of an unconscious differs from that of the neurotic. The psychotic chooses the foreclosure of the Name-of-the-Father, and the implication of this first choice is the short-circuiting of the (lawful) functioning of the unconscious as such. Because the psychotic, by definition, does not choose the signifier (S1), I argue that we must reconsider what is truly at stake for the psychotic in the face of a *second* choice.

Whether or not the subject of psychosis initially "chooses her unconscious" remains an open and an extremely important question. To choose the unconscious is to submit to the law of language and thus to receive the protection of the signifier. Nonetheless, what is compelling about Zupancic's formulation is the insistence upon the "possibility of choice" and its return. Of interest here are the particular stakes of the return of choice (and "freedom") for the psychotic.

The psychotic's perception of the rupture, and the absence of the Good, as "evil", is the background against which the problem of the second choice, and the introduction of desire itself, is set. As I note earlier, the *act* is initially perceived as evil from the perspective of psychotic certainty. If we follow Zupancic a bit further we can clarify this question at the level of ideological structure and its limit. She writes: "It is a matter of acknowledging that any ethical act, precisely insofar as it is an act, is necessarily 'evil'" (p. 95). We must distinguish "empirical evil" from that which is inherent to the structure of the act:

> This is the evil that belongs to the very structure of the act, to the fact that the latter always implies a 'transgression', a change in 'what is'. (p. 95)

As with the relation of delusion to dream, we are interested in the structural relation between *ideology* and the ethical *act*. I situate psychotic delusion on the side of 'ideology' (Fig. 6.2).

The source of the act will emerge from the dream in order to contest the delusion and, ultimately, *externalize* the object (the voice). It is from

```
Ideology/delusion <------------ act/dream
--------------------            --------------
internal voice/object ----------> lacking object
```

Fig. 6.2 Structural relation between ideology and the ethical act

the position of ideological certainty that the psychotic will perceive the lack in the dream as evil, i.e., the lacking object *acting in the dream* comes from a scene that is radically Other to the certainty of delusion and the delusion's aim of maintaining an ideology capable of completely excluding the lack. From the perspective of certainty the act can only be perceived as "evil": thus the act (the "gap", or thing "out-of-place") is recognized here only as the rupture itself, nothing more. The act (the emergence of a gap) requires the risk of a second choice.

In other words, as I suggest earlier, the ethical choice is precisely the choice to enter into the space opened up by the rupture.

Whether or not to enter that space is the ethical choice put to the psychotic by the lack in the dream—a lack that is at odds with the ideological project of delusion. This is a delicate point in the installation of the transference where—and this is my hypothesis—the rupture (its potential) may persist in juxtaposition with the certainty of delusion. In other words, that a rupture/lack enters into the psychotic's discourse of delusion does not necessarily imply that she will answer to the lack and produce a new speech that is 'of' the subject. The analyst's desire (as support for the field of ethics) comes into play at this point.

6.8.2 The Subject Is a Question

This brings us full circle to where I introduced my patient with his question "Do you think there is any truth to it [to my theory]?". His question seemed to function as a response of the subject (unconscious) provoked both by the analyst's desire to know and by the subsequent dream-work. What this patient called his "theory" was in fact a part of his delusion. In brief, the theory consisted in the patient's "belief" that, because he made more money than his father, he would, in turn, "have more children than his father and marry a woman more beautiful than his mother". He continued: "This is a theory *we* have … do you think there is any truth to it."

As with the previous example, I simply want to underscore the way in which the field of the dream yielded memories and then, most importantly, a question that is at odds with the aim of his delusion. With his question regarding the "theory" he, for the first time in the course of the treatment, says something that betrays that he is not certain of himself. He must now face the stakes of his question as such. In other words, his *question* functions as a subversive force with the potential effect of undermining delusional certainty. Until this point in the treatment he had been grappling with questions coming from the analyst, for example, questions aimed either at the content of the voice, to evoke the dream, or to support the elaboration of the dream-work. While the analyst's question (desire) has proved productive in provoking dreams and associative material, the hazard is always that the analyst's question/desire will be perceived by the psychotic as persecutory and, ultimately, produce paranoia on the side of the psychotic versus transference defined as a desire-to-know.

The fundamental importance of his question is that it marks an instance of a desire-to-know (a lack-of-knowing) on the side of the psychotic. The consequence of the emergence of his question is that, henceforward, he has a choice to either pursue the *question* (his desire) or to continue his efforts to shore up the delusion.

6.9 The Analyst's Desire and Act: A New Guarantee for the Psychotic

As we confront the question of *ethics without ethics* we must also confront the problem of a *guarantee without guarantee*. The new guarantee issues from the status of the desire in play—a desire designed to provoke the transference defined as a desire for unconscious knowledge. In *Seminar XI* Lacan says the following of the analyst's desire:

> The analyst's desire is not a pure desire. It is a desire to obtain absolute difference, a desire which intervenes when, confronted with the primary signifier, the subject is, for the first time, in a position to subject himself to it. (p. 276)

This is a conception of desire-as-support for the subject.

The analyst must act to take the position of a witness, and a support, for the process of confrontation with the failure of the universal that "returns" with the emergence of the rupture. The act of the analyst (as witness to the experience of absence) exists, and functions, only in relation to the problem of the said absence of a Good, or guarantee. In *Seminar VII*, Lacan links the problem of the absence of a Good to the action of the analyst.

> The question of the Sovereign Good is one that man has asked himself since time immemorial. But the analyst knows that it is a question that is closed. Not only doesn't he [the analyst] have that Sovereign Good that is asked of him, but he also knows there isn't any. (p. 300)

A correct apprehension of what the analyst *knows* (the "analyst's desire") is integral to forming an understanding of the transference as, to use psychoanalyst Willy Apollon's term, an "ethical fulcrum". Lacan Continues:

> What the analyst has to give, unlike the partner in the act of love … is … what he has. And what he has is nothing other than his desire, like that of the analysand, with the difference that it is an experienced desire. (p. 300)

What does the analyst have to offer the psychotic in her confrontation with the void? The analyst's offering (an "experienced desire") consists precisely in the knowledge that there is no Sovereign Good from which the subject might derive Happiness or total satisfaction. In other words, the analyst offers the lack of such a guarantee, which is the analyst's desire to know the subject's experience of, and solutions to, absence—and lack itself. It is from the position of a *learned ignorance* (desire/lack), in the face of the subject's experience of the absence of the Good, that the analyst maintains an ethical position vis-à-vis the subject of the unconscious.

So, we have a guarantee, embodied in the analyst's desire, that offers the possibility of living without the tyranny of the Good.

What does this last formulation tell us about the relation of psychoanalysis to the Law? Situating the analyst's action in the field of the letter implies that the analyst is not on the side of the Law *per se*, but that the analyst (necessarily with the psychotic) acts in an ethical field beyond the limits of the Law, a field that, because it is beyond the Law (as pure command or social 'Ideal'), is by definition an ethics of the body (and of death drive). Although the psychotic, under transference, may come to terms with the lack or *truth* in the Law, she will necessarily do so without the Good and without the social Ideals that protect the neurotic.

The ethical status of the analyst's desire is the only guarantee for the psychotic that the analyst is on her side. Apollon (1991) argues that the analyst contests the psychotic's position as 'object' from "under the law of the letter and writing", thus indicating a notion of a *law of the letter* that is outside, or on the *Other side*, of the Law of Language (p. 137). Apollon's intervention is important in that he suggests a "law of the letter" that is set in contrast to the Sense conferred by the signifier (S1). So, the desire (ethic) of the analyst is situated in line with the *letter* (object a), the *body*, and the *Voice*. In other words, the analyst's desire follows the *truth* of the Law—a truth that is revealed only when the Law is stripped of its Ideals. It is in this sense that we can understand Lacan's conception of the analyst's desire as an "experienced" desire, such that the analyst's desire is founded on the knowledge (*savoir*) of the inadequacy of the signifier and the lack in the Law.

It is the responsibility of the analyst not to abuse the psychotic by taking the side of the Ideals, of Sense, or of Biology. The psychotic already knows that the limits offered by the Ideals and Biology have failed and she will require the analyst to offer a different way. Like the psychotic, the analyst finds his or her ethic where all other limits fail. With recourse only to his or her own *savoir* of the Other's lack and its effects, the analyst offers the psychotic a new way to put the drive to work, and to call forth the subject through the dream.

6.10 Conclusion: Becoming a Subject of (the Truth in) the Moral Law

Does the psychotic's choice to speak, and to answer the call of the unconscious, constitute the emergence of the subject of desire itself from the closed universe of psychosis? In other words, does the psychotic, in contrast to the neurotic, face its (first) *division* (its *Spaltung*) under transference? If so, this would explain why we must take a different path to engage the psychotic in the analytic experience and in the provocation of a desire to know the truth of the Law.

The fact that this question remains open is significant. Lacan's definition of the analyst's desire, quoted earlier, says as much about the stakes for the subject (faced with a choice) as it does about the status, and function, of the analyst's desire. The analyst's desire intervenes, as support, where the subject "confronted with the primary signifier" is "for the first time, in a position to subject himself to it" (p. 276). The "primary signifier", in other words the primary *effects* of the signifier (lack), is brought back into play vis-à-vis the analyst's desire to know. In the case under discussion the analyst's desire evoked a question on the side of the patient. I contend that his question functions as a reintroduction (or perhaps introduction) of lack into his experience. In this case, his *question* is functioning as the subject as such. The subject, as a gap or question mark, functions to bore a hole in delusion.

The signifier, the Law, is required for the advent of the subject of psychoanalysis. The point is to support the psychotic's confrontation with the signifier in the least cruel way possible. The analyst achieves this (lack of cruelty) by contesting cruelty as such, and by joining the psychotic in an ethical field that opens beyond the limit set by the Good (and Evil).

References

Apollon, W. (1991). Theory and practice in the psychoanalytic practice of psychosis. In E. Ragland-Sullivan & M. Bracher (Eds.), *Lacan and the subject of language* (pp. 116–140). Routledge.

Apollon, et. al. (2002). *After Lacan: Clinical practice and the subject of the unconscious.* (Eds.), R. Hughes & K.R. Malone New York: SUNY Press.

Aristotle. (1975). *Nichomachean ethics* (M. Ostwald, Trans.). The Bobbs Merrill Co., Inc.

Deleuze, G., & Guattari, F. (1983). *Anti-Oedipus: Capitalism and Schizophrenia.* University of Minnesota Press.

Deleuze, G., & Guattari, F. (1987). How do you make yourself a body without organs? In *A thousand plateaus: capitalism and schizophrenia* (pp. 149–166). University of Minnesota Press.

Kant, I. (1788) (1956). *The critique of practical reason* (L.W. Beck, Trans.). Macmillan Publishing Co.
Lacan, J. (1978). *The four fundamental concepts of psychoanalysis, the seminar of Jacques Lacan, Book XI* (J.A. Miller, Ed., A. Sheridan, Trans.). W.W. Norton & Co.
Lacan, J. (1992). *The ethics of psychoanalysis (1959–1960), The seminar of Jacques Lacan, Book VII* (J.A. Miller, Ed., D. Porter, Trans.). W.W. Norton & Co.
Lacan, J. (1993). *The psychoses (1955–1956), The seminar of Jacques Lacan, Book III* (J.A. Miller, Ed., R. Grigg, Trans.). W.W. Norton & Co.
Lacan, J. (2006). Kant with Sade. In *Ecrits: the first complete edition in English* (B. Fink, Ed., and Trans.). New York: W.W. Norton and Co.
MacCannell, J. F. (2000). *The Hysteric's guide to the future female subject.* University of Minnesota Press.
Zupancic, A. (2000). *Ethics of the real: Kant, Lacan.* Verso.

7

The Fear of Psychosis: Part I

7.1 The Hearing Voices Movement: What Do People with Lived Experience Have to Teach Clinicians?

Operating from a place of fear leads to clinical approaches that stigmatize and punish those who have extreme experiences. All that I have discussed thus far is within the limits of a one-on-one analytic model. However, the most successful approaches to psychosis are those that include multiple pathways for the expression and understanding of extreme experiences. Therefore we will now turn towards another approach to understanding and intervening in psychosis that was founded by people with a lived experience of psychosis. The Hearing Voices Network (HVN) has much to teach clinicians about being courageous and respectful in the face of extreme experiences. My hope is that engaging with the HVN can help guide clinicians to be more inclusive and respectful of psychotic experiences and to invent new ways to create vital connections and trust with people experiencing psychosis.

It is well known that the HVN peer-facilitated groups provide support and a sense of community to people with lived experience of psychosis.

B. Fimiani, *Psychosis and Extreme States*, The Palgrave Lacan Series,
https://doi.org/10.1007/978-3-030-75440-2_7

However, in my experience collaborating with the San Francisco Bay Area HVN, and in discussions with voice hearers/peers within the organization, I have observed that the work internal to the Hearing Voices (HV) groups advances beyond offering only 'support' and constitutes a form of treatment. In this chapter I will discuss how the HV groups are, spontaneously in my view, developing a way to effectively 'treat' persistent psychotic phenomena including 'distressing beliefs' (aka "delusions" in clinical terms) and disturbing voices. I am a Board member of the San Francisco Bay Area HVN and I work closely with members of the organization to promote our mission and to create new HV groups. I am thus aware that my use of the word 'treatment' with regard to HV groups is at odds with the stated aims of the HVN. Within the HVN the term treatment is understood to further pathologize voice hearing given that the term 'treatment' evokes the need for an 'illness' to be 'treated'. The principles and the Charter of the HVN state that voice hearing is not to be understood, solely, as deriving from illness.

As I intend to argue that the HV groups produce a form of treatment, I will take a moment here to contextualize and justify my use of the term 'treatment'. My use of the term treatment necessarily follows from how I have thus far defined the meaning of the term "symptom", such that my use of the term treatment is intended as non-stigmatizing. For example, in earlier chapters of this book I have separated the term symptom from the medical model. The definition of the term symptom within the medical model identifies phenomena such as voices or disturbing thoughts as symptoms of an underlying 'disease' and therefore as phenomena to be suppressed or eradicated. Thus 'treatment' within the medical model, whether as a pharmacological, behavioural, or psychological intervention, aims to achieve the goal of simply reducing or stopping the occurrence of the symptom.

In contrast, my clinical approach views the symptom in a very different light. In psychoanalytic terms the symptom is understood as a metaphor and as analysts we suppose that the symptom contains important knowledge for the person experiencing psychosis. Therefore in my psychoanalytic model the term 'treatment' suggests a method designed to support the person experiencing psychosis in 'decoding' the symptom with the aim of revealing the knowledge that the symptom contains. It is in the spirit of discovery (of knowledge), and the creation of insight and opportunities for change, that I use the term treatment. I have found that the HV groups also approach psychotic experiences ("symptoms") with a similar ethic of curiosity and with a desire to support people in discovering the context and meaning of their experiences. I will discuss similarities and differences between my psychoanalytic approach to psychosis and the mechanisms of change working within the HV groups. In both approaches there is a 'symbolic' treatment of delusion and distressing voices but the 'technique' used by the respective approaches is of course different. However, the 'ethical position' taken up by the analyst or peer in relation to psychotic speech is similar.

The HVM was founded in the 1980s in reaction to the stigmatizing effect of the mental health system. The presence of the HVN around the globe involves international, national, and regional organizations that all share a common purpose. For example, *Inter-Voice* is the title of the international manifestation of the HVN. The following description can be found on the *Inter-voice* website:

> The International Hearing Voices Movement consists of the diverse conversations, initiatives, groups and individuals around the world that share some core values. These include: hearing voices, seeing visions and related phenomena are meaningful experiences that can be understood in many ways; hearing voices is not, in itself, an indication of illness—but difficulties coping with voices can cause great distress; when people are overwhelmed by their experiences, support offered should be based on respect, empathy, informed choice and an understanding of the personal meaning voices have in someone's life.
>
> As a movement of diverse people, countries and ideas, we recognise the importance of hearing and including many voices. As such beside our basic values we do not speak with one voice. We welcome multiple perspectives and ways of contributing. Change can happen on an individual, group, community and societal level—so whether you are working towards making sense of your own voice hearing experience, sharing information in your social circles, trying to improve the support on offer to others or are creating systemic change—we welcome you. (Inter-Voice: The International Hearing Voices Network, 2021, http://www.intervoiceonline.org)

My discussion in this chapter will revolve around an interview with a person with lived experience of psychosis who is a member and educator within the HVM. The following is the transcript of the interview. At particular nodal points in the interview I will depart from the transcript to discuss how the interviewee provides insight into the function of fear in the mental health system. In the same fashion, at particular moments in the transcript, I will discuss how the interviewee's experience and examples from group processes reveal, in my assessment, how treatment is taking place in the HVN group setting. My commentary will be marked with the headings "Editorial note" or "Conceptual Interlude".

7.2 The Fear of Psychosis: Interview with Peer-specialist and Educator Cindy Marty Hadge

I met Cindy Marty Hadge when she came to San Francisco to conduct an HV group facilitator training with our clinical team. Cindy is an exceptional human being, a gifted educator and group facilitator, and the story of her recovery has provided hope to many.

The following biographical information is in Cindy's own words:

Cindy is a person who experienced physical, emotional, sexual and medical trauma as a child. She experienced voices, visions and thoughts of ending her [life] while growing up. As a young adult she turned to alcohol and street drugs in an effort to make life livable. Over time she entered the mental health system, where the street drugs were replaced with prescribed drugs and the result was frequently the same—walking or stumbling through life in a mind-numbing state and while continuing to experience voices, visions and thoughts of ending her life.

Knowing that peer support in the form of 12 Step programs had been helpful in her struggling with substance use, she sought out peer support for her emotional distress and experience of extreme states. Cindy discovered that she lived within walking distance of one of the Western Mass Recovery Learning Community (WMRLC) […] spaces, where one of the very few Hearing Voices Network (HVN) groups in the US was held. Within the WMRLC […] she found healing and hope. By attending HVN groups she discovered that there were things she could do beyond taking medication to navigate her experience.

Currently Cindy has found the meaning, purpose and connection that she longed for and has made a way of making sense of the senseless and is transforming her tragedies into treasures by being healed when creating space for others to heal. Cindy is gender non-conforming and has presented both as Cindy and Marty. Cindy is a keynote speaker and a national trainer.

Prior to the interview with Cindy I sent her the following questions to guide our conversation on the topic of the 'fear of psychosis': Do you think fear on the side of the clinician affects how clinicians interact with (listen to) a person experiencing psychosis? Do you think that there is a lack of curiosity, amongst clinicians of various disciplines, about what people with psychosis have to say? Do you think there is something that the person experiencing psychosis 'knows' that society does not want to know? Finally, how can the principles of the Hearing Voices Movement teach clinicians to be better listeners when working with voice hearers that are in distress?

When I attended Cindy's group facilitator training in 2018, I was struck by how a peer-run group model had discovered a way of listening, and 'questioning' participant narratives, which in turn could lead participants to challenge long-standing fixed and disturbing belief systems. Cindy refers to participants' belief systems as "frameworks" versus the term used by mental health clinicians, i.e., 'delusion'. There is a clear parallel between the clinical-ethical approach that I have discussed in the previous chapters of this book and the approach that people with lived experience have discovered while working together in groups. In particular, I suggest that there is a parallel between the way 'delusion' is contested and treated in my clinical model and the ways that 'thought systems' (aka delusions or what Cindy terms "frameworks") are challenged and 'treated' through the spontaneous work, between peers, in the HV groups. I will discuss this parallel after we hear from Cindy directly.

Cindy began one of our discussions by explaining her use of the term "framework" and in particular how the HV group process, guided by curiosity and genuine interest, can lead a participant to discover deeply personal issues that underlie the persistence of disturbing beliefs and voices.

Cindy Marty Hadge (CMH):

The *framework* is the way in which somebody tries to make sense of what's going on for them. So somebody's framework might be, for example, "I was abducted by aliens". Or somebody's framework might be "I have a chemical imbalance" or "I'm having a spiritual experience".[1] So there are lots of different ways that people try to make sense of what they're going through.

Bret Fimiani (BF):

You just said that one 'framework' might be "I have a chemical imbalance". So it seems that the medical model ("chemical imbalance") is also considered a 'framework', that is, a way one might make sense of a psychotic experience?

CMH:

Correct, and within the Hearing Voices Movement, all frameworks are accepted. People get to determine what framework makes sense to them. And over time somebody's framework may *change* and it may change many times. But ideally we are neutral on whatever a person's framework is and our job is to, if the person is interested, explore that with them. We might ask, "How does that work?" or "How does that work in your world?"

So, there was a person I met in a [Hearing Voices] group who would keep going through a different framework, like every month. One month it was about cockroaches—the voices were coming from cockroaches. One month the voices were coming from the TV, or radio, or from electricity. Another time it [voice and belief system] was about animals. The voices were coming from animals. But you know, maybe a year, a year and a half into the group, once we could deal with the content of the voices—and it took a while for the person to get to that place—they realized that what this was really about was being sexually abused by a priest and all the shame and guilt they had about that. But it wasn't until that person felt safe enough, or validated enough, or believed enough, or built

[1] Note that, although I use the term 'psychosis' through this book, Cindy herself does not use the term psychosis to describe or categorize her personal experience. She clarified with me that, rather than psychosis, she tends to use the term "spiritual experience" to refer to her various inner experiences.

trust, that the person could talk about this without being judged, assessed or labelled—they realize, "I can just be met with curiosity". It took a while, but once they got to this place, they could then talk about the content of the voices. And that's when they started to be able to put the pieces together. I actually knew six months into the group that the person's themes were themes of somebody who had been sexually abused. *But they needed to come to that understanding on their own.* Do you know what I mean?

BF: You had a sense that there was a theme of abuse underlying their voices and beliefs?

CMH:

Yeah, because of the things that they were wrestling with. One idea they had for a solution was that they needed to stop masturbating. So to me, that was all their shame and guilt wrapped up with this. So yeah, there are themes that come up frequently with people who have been sexually abused, and this person was expressing those themes.

BF:

Now, I imagine that for you, the ability to hear the themes—to know the themes—comes from many years of listening?

CMH:

Well, many years of listening and also from my own lived experience. It is amazing to meet people from other countries, all over this world, and there are themes that come up frequently. You know, it's not exactly the same themes from person to person, but so many of the feelings that people wrestle with are pretty common.

BF:

With the person you have been discussing, the voices were being explained by various frameworks. I'm struck that this person went from framework to framework to framework. They did not just stick with one framework?

CMH:

No, they were trying to make sense of it—the voices and beliefs. They would come to group and they would have this idea, "this is what's going on". And we would talk about that and what that could mean? You know, if this is what's going on, what are the things that you can do to feel more comfortable in the world? And they would try different things. And so we brainstormed together in the group. And so the person unplugged everything at night or covered things with a blanket so the voices wouldn't be so loud. And then we'd go on to a different framework because this framework was not working for them.

BF: That's what I was wondering. Shifting from one framework to another seems to suggest that a given framework was no longer working—as a 'solution'—and that there was a type of work happening in the group. It seems that your curiosity about [and questioning of] the particular framework would lead that person to reach the limit of a particular framework and then they would create a new framework.

CMH:

Right, absolutely.

BF:

And, over the course of a year and a half, eventually, there was this kind of travelling from frameworks to his or her traumatic history. Is this right?

CMH:

Right. And so there's also this thing that happens. People will sometimes come into the group and give you something like the 'police report', for example, "This happened and then this happened and then this happened". To actually get to, "*What did it feel like? What did it make you think? How do you understand that?*" These questions sometimes don't get addressed. Or, for example, if a crisis clinician asks me if I'm "hearing voices", and I say yes, then they'll say, "Are they 'commanding' voices or are they telling you to 'hurt' yourself or somebody else?" And that's usually the final question on the voices [from a clinician]. They [clinicians] don't ask, "What does it remind you of? Is there a metaphor? Is there a context?" That's all missing. And so somebody might come to the group who's received a lot of [mental health] services and they're used to just saying what their "symptoms" are, and not really talking about, for example, "when does it [voices and beliefs] come, and in relationship to what?" The context of the voices is frequently left out of any discussion with clinicians.

7.2.1 Conceptual Interlude: A Common Ethic

I agree that Cindy's stance is 'neutral' in that she does not intend to directly contest the truth of anyone's framework. However, I suggest that the curiosity, expressed through questioning, is quite active and driven by a desire to understand the meaning or 'logic' of a particular person's explanation of their experience. Cindy's approach is similar, in its ethic of respect and curiosity, to the way I have described the analyst's position with regard to the speech of a person experiencing psychosis. Thus one similarity between the analytic and HVN approaches is that both approaches begin with an ethic of respect and curiosity, and both approaches operate with the premise that voices and belief systems (delusions or "frameworks") are inherently meaningful to the person experiencing psychosis. This premise stands in contrast to the approaches deployed within contemporary psychiatry and many psychological approaches that operate with the basic assumption that psychotic phenomena stem from a brain disease, and/or represent a failure to align oneself with consensual reality.

A second similarity between the analytic and HVN approaches is evident in the anecdote that Cindy described earlier regarding how the group process led a member to "change" their framework. What is the engine or cause of the change of framework in her example? Cindy describes a process in the HV group where she and other members ask questions about the framework and in essence encourage the person to explain how the framework 'works' or functions for them. As Cindy says earlier, the member may change frameworks because a given framework is 'no longer working for them'. The aim of the HV group is to explore a given framework asking such questions as *"how does that work … what did it feel like … when did you first hear or see that"*? Cindy clarified that the phenomenon of "changing frameworks" is a common occurrence in HV groups. Furthermore, following Cindy's example, the changing of frameworks is preliminary to a possible discovery of an underlying subjective and traumatic history that a given framework has been designed to explain, for example, where the person in Cindy's example arrived at the realization that her voices and distressing beliefs corresponded to her history "of being abused by a priest".

Importantly, Cindy observed that the group member "needed to come to that understanding on their own". So here we have a technique ('questioning' of the framework/delusion) and an underlying ethic that are common to both the analytic and HV approaches. One difference in technique is that, in the analytic approach that I have outlined in earlier chapters, the clinician explicitly uses the dream-work to facilitate the emergence of new knowledge on the side of the patient. Yet the ethical stance in both approaches requires that the clinician and the HV group peer-facilitator understand that any new knowledge must come from *within* the person experiencing psychosis. In both the HV and analytic approaches the 'contestation' (challenging) of psychotic belief systems is understood to originate from within the person and never from the analyst or peer facilitator. I believe that this fundamental and shared ethical stance makes it more likely that any new knowledge (e.g., the member's linking of voices to traumatic history) will be accepted as credible by the person experiencing psychosis.

Returning to the interview

Cindy and I next discussed her experience of going through a crisis in a hospital setting versus going through a crisis in a "peer respite centre".[2] Whereas in the hospital she found that she was often over-medicated and stripped of personal responsibility and agency, in the peer respite centre she found less emphasis on medicating (suppressing) the crisis and rather the opportunity to go through the crisis in connection with peer-specialists who could be genuinely curious about her experience. She noted that the hospital environment would often compound her trauma

[2] For readers who may be unfamiliar with the peer respite model: Typically the term peer respite refers to a residence staffed by non-clinicians trained as peer-specialists, that is, people with lived experience of psychosis or extreme states that are in recovery and have been formally trained to support someone experiencing a crisis. Peer respites are intended as safe places where a person in crisis can reside for, typically, up to one week while they pass through a crisis. By design, peer respites are intended as an alternative to hospitalization. "Afiya", a program of the WMRLC, is one such peer respite. Per the WMRLC website (2021), "Afiya strives to provide a safe place in which each person can find the balance and support needed to turn what is so often referred to as a 'crisis' into a growth and learning opportunity."

while the peer respite did not. Cindy began by discussing the often-traumatic effects of hospitalization.

CMH:

The thing that is so troubling so many times is that forced commitment brings up the issue of trauma. You're powerless, at least [in my experience] they're going to tell you [to] take off your clothes and they take everything away and you can't communicate with anyone, you know. In my experience which is not everybody's experience, generally it might be *gang restraint*, which is, if you are a survivor of sexual trauma, having somebody take away your clothes and strap you to a bed is a pretty shitty event. You are replicating that trauma, for example, [hospital staff may imply] *"if you don't take off your clothes and put on this Johnny, we have these guys who are going to come in and help you do it"*. So any personal boundaries or personal agency can get lost.

Editorial Note:

Cindy had recently given the keynote address at the 2019 National Conference of the International Society for Psychological and Social Approaches to Psychosis (ISPS) in New Haven, CT, where she discussed how messages that, for her, may have originated with traumatic events (various forms of abuse) and later manifested in negative voices and thoughts were often "echoed" by the approach of mental health clinicians in hospital settings.

In her ISPS conference presentation Cindy presented the parallel messages in the following way:

Messages that can come with Trauma

- Don't tell or someone will get hurt.
- They won't believe you anyway.
- They will say you are crazy.
- Quit fighting and make it easier on yourself.
- I am doing this for your own good.
- You should be grateful you have it this good.

In comparison to:

Messages often found in Clinical Settings

- If you talk about it, you can lose your rights.
- Your experiences are not real.
- You are mentally ill.
- Be compliant or it will get worse.
- We are doing this for your own good.
- Accept and be happy with a very limited life.

The result: Mental Health services may *ECHO* the past trauma rather than addressing it.

Reinforcing feelings and experiences of:

- Powerlessness
- Shame and guilt
- Silencing
- Impending doom
- Hopelessness
- And sometimes forcing capitulation to authority[3]

Cindy's observation highlights how negative messages from medical and mental health providers can echo and thus confirm negative messages that come from sources of abuse and from one's voices and distressing thoughts.

CMH:

In contrast, when I went to the [peer] respite, the first thing they [peer-staff] said to me was "What can we do to help?" Initially this freaked me out because I was like "*oh, my God if you don't know what to do … I actually don't know what to do!*" But what was really great about it [peer approach] was it put some responsibility back into my hands. I was given the opportunity and the belief that I might have some wisdom about *me* and *my experience. I could then get over the idea that, "Oh I want someone to rescue me or fix it*".

Another problem I would have going to the hospital is that they used to have this thing where they would have me lie down in a bed and I

[3] Hadge, C.M. (2019, October 14–17). *Living in the Margins and the Struggle to Reclaim Citizenship* [Paper presentation]. ISPS-US National Conference, New Haven, Connecticut, USA.

really didn't want to. I spent many, many years of my life not being able to sleep in a bed. I can sleep on a sofa but not in a bed. This makes sense in terms of the trauma I went through. But nobody was really curious about that when I was in a locked unit. They just saw that [not wanting to lie in a bed] as "*you're being stubborn*" or whatever they thought. But at the respite I could sleep on the floor, turn out all the lights, put on headphones, and eventually my system would calm down.

The psychiatrist I had at the time—he used a number of metaphors which I didn't like—but then he used this one, "*it's like you're a computer and you have too many windows open and you're locking up*". So his pitch was if you go to the hospital and we put you on medication it will help you "reboot". It [medication] will stop everything, which it would. It would stop everything. [At the respite] I got a chance to do that on my own, just to stop everything.

What was awesome about the respite too was that I could feel that I was not alone. And that there was no requirement of me to participate or communicate in a certain way. A couple [of] things happened when I was there. There was one night where in the middle of the night I had a moment of *clarity and presence* and I said to the person [peer] working there: "Do you plan on sleeping tonight or can I talk with you?" Instead of being sent to bed or told to stay in my room or give[n] a shot of medication there was this person there I could talk to. I had that moment of time where someone could understand what I was saying and we could have a conversation.

BF:

And Cindy, was that a peer that you had the conversation with?

CMH:

Well it was someone working at the respite and everybody working there has gone through their own self-described experiences. He was somebody trained for Intentional Peer Support.

So, another example, one night I was there I felt like I wasn't totally out of my crisis that I was going through, but I also didn't want to be alone. In my mind I felt like I might just disappear. I needed to feel somehow connected. But I wasn't able to have a conversation, at least not one that somebody else could understand. It was maybe four o'clock in the morning I started putting together the ping-pong table in the basement.

Somebody came down and we did it together and we didn't talk. Occasionally we'd look at the directions and give each other things. We spent hours doing it and *that was peer support … that was someone being with me.*

I will say that there was at least one time where I thought "I can try to ride this out on my own or ride this out without a lot of psych drugs [in hospital]". But I made a decision that I'd rather do the psych drugs—I was at this place where I just wanted this to stop. I would say it would be awesome if people had a choice and to know there was an option to not necessarily do psych drugs and have a choice regarding what kind of support they want.

BF:

A question about your psychiatrist's 'rebooting' metaphor: It sounds like that was a somewhat useful metaphor to you. For you, how does rebooting via medication compare to say rebooting via the peer respite model?

CMH:

Oh, for me it's better without the medication because things come back in a natural order whereas if I went into the hospital, and they put me on Thorazine or Haldol, things come back slowly and in a mishmash way. It would take me much longer. If I go to the hospital I'm probably going to take those things [medications] for two weeks and stop. They will have served their purpose. I'm not into this belief system that you need to be on them for a long time and, in fact, the longer I'm on them the harder it is to get off them. I mean literally if I'm on medication I can't read, I can't think, I can't formulate coherent thoughts or I might get a thought and, if I pause, I lose it. So medication actually slows everything—including recovery.

BF:

Okay, so without medication and in the peer respite things come back in a more linear way or a more orderly way?

CMH:

For me, for lack of a better word, in a more natural way. The things that are really important or really core come back first.

BF:

Do you have an example of what it means that "things come back to you in a natural way"?

CMH:

So, I can remember my supervisor at Western Mass Recovery Learning Community was calling me in the hospital and saying, "You have a training next week. … Caroline just wants to know if you're going to get out of the hospital in time to do it". I said: "Yes by next week I will be able to do that." So what was important to me was to be able to do the trainings. What was important to me was to be connected to my community. Even if I wasn't fully back, I could be back enough to be fully present for the training. Maybe not for any other part of the day, but I knew I would have enough wherewithal and the energy to do that.

Or, another way to look at this is: if I'm in a place where nothing seems real or I can't trust anything or if I don't even know what is real and what is not … what would come back first for me, without medication, would be the things I believe are important. At one point in my life before HVN I would carry a notebook and in it I would write down things that I heard or I read that I just believed were core beliefs like "I have a right to say no or I'm not responsible for other people's feelings". Then when I had so many other voices and thoughts and things that were getting in the way I could look in the book and put these grounding messages into my head. So those are the things that would come back first.

Many people learn how to go through the motions to get out of the hospital, but it wouldn't be like I was grounded or actually had hope or anything. It's just more like "okay, I just need to get out of hospital now so I need to figure out what it is I'm supposed to say so I can get out".

BF:

Versus, for example, when your training director called you at the hospital and said: "Are you ready for your training?" And you said "Yeah I'll be ready." That was not going through the motions?

CMH:

Yes and plus it was this totally different perspective [from training director] of "I have faith in you moving through this". She's reminding me who I am and what I'm capable of. Just a positive belief that somebody can move through something versus a fear that they can't or they're going to decompensate or whatever. Versus, just asking "are you stable?", which is what they might ask me at the hospital.

BF:

Versus a psychiatric re-evaluation where often a clinician is not going to address you in that way.

CMH:

Frequently people in clinical roles are working under the false assumption that somehow they are *responsible for* other people and that they can predict what's going to happen.

Editorial Note:

In a previous discussion with Cindy she discussed the difference between being "responsible for" and "responsible to" someone experiencing psychosis. We return to this distinction in the latter part of this interview. In short, the term being 'responsible for' implies that the clinician does not allow the person experiencing psychosis to discover their solutions on their own, whereas the term being 'responsible to' implies a stance where the clinician or peer-specialist attempts *only* to facilitate a process of discovery on the side of the person experiencing psychosis, as in Cindy's earlier example of the group member's discovery of the theme underlying their voices and distressing beliefs.

CMH:

So if I'm a clinician and sitting here saying I need to err on the side of *my safety*, *my liability*, and *my employment*, then I'm not going to have faith or take a risk about this person. I'm going to be very conservative. For example, I can remember having my outreach worker at the Department of Mental Health Services come and see me and tell me how "wonderful" I was doing. I said: "I have no life. I don't get off my sofa. I smoke cigarettes, drink coffee and watch TV all day." She's like "You're doing wonderful, you're not getting into any trouble."

BF: Such that, 'You're stable … you are not getting into trouble.'

CMH:

Yeah, so their idea of recovery is limited and their job is to keep me even, or 'flat'. What was different with Sera Davidow [supervisor] and the Western Mass Recovery Learning Community was that my recovery went fast. I would try all these new things and then hit a wall, then dip down and hopefully I would learn something and then I would build back up and go further along in my recovery—at least that's been my experience.

With voices, it's a standard clinical approach to say the voices are 'not real', and to ignore them or deny them. But how am I ever going to figure it out without looking at it? When is denial a good strategy? How am I ever going to learn how to navigate the experience if I spent all my time trying to pretend it's not happening? If I'm not looking at my experience close enough how am I going to figure out what is happening with my experience, and in relationship to what?

BF:

Can you share your metaphor about "being followed on the street"? It seems to be a good metaphor for what we are discussing now on the topic of the denial, or suppression, of voices versus taking a more curious or investigative stance towards the voices.

CMH:

Right, that was huge for me. So I go into the hearing voices group and it's *not* about 'how to make the voices stop', and so I'm irritated. I was like "I thought you're going to teach me how *not* to have voices". So anyway, Gail Hornstein started asking me questions. Gail was one of the group facilitators and she is the Mount Holyoke College Professor who wrote "Agnes's Jackets". I really didn't talk much then. When I first went to the group I was on Thorazine so I wasn't a big talker anyhow. But eventually, maybe six months in, she finally said something that made sense to me. She said: "You're walking down the street and someone is walking behind you. You cross the street and they cross the street. Then you start walking faster and they start walking faster and maybe you start running and then they start running." Then Gail said: *"Sometimes there's a value to turning around and asking them, what do you want?"* So that made sense to me and I said: "Well maybe I do need to look at what I'm going through or maybe I do need to talk about what the voices are saying. Maybe I need to look at my experience."

But I had all those years in the mental health system where I was told not to look at my experience and that recovery involved not having or denying the voices versus learning how to navigate *with* them. It was like a big paradigm shift that I needed to go through.

Editorial Note: Next Cindy and I discussed how curiosity and responsibility are linked in the HV group model.

BF:

I also wanted to ask you about the quality of your curiosity, for example, with regard [to] the person that we discussed earlier in the HV group with multiple and changing "frameworks". You noted that you could hear the 'themes'; however, you didn't impose your concept of a theme on the member. Your curiosity stayed very close to what the person was saying. Is that something you have to negotiate within yourself, being sure to sideline your own hypotheses, so that you can remain truly curious?

CMH:

So what I try to do is check for understanding. I'll say: "Well, this is what I'm hearing. Is it like this or is it like that?" I love it, I love trying to be open to hearing, because sometimes people have words that describe something I've felt or wrestled with or went through. And they have insight or words that just explain something in me, and that's a gift. It's a gift to hear their perspective, so I am honestly curious. Or sometimes, when I check for understanding, somebody will say: "Oh no. It was not like that at all. You don't know at all. You don't understand." And I would say: "You're right, explain it to me … I'm trying really hard to understand and I *don't* get it. So please, help me. Help me to understand."

7.2.2 Conceptual Interlude: The Position of the Listener, and Questioning Delusion with HVN and Psychoanalysis

Here we have another similarity between the analytic approach and the HVN approach to someone experiencing voices and distressing beliefs. In this case, the similarity regards the position of the listener and the method of questioning delusion. As I have discussed in earlier chapters of this book, the position of the analyst (as listener) is key to successful engagement with a person experiencing psychosis. Cindy's stance of 'non-knowing', and of supposing the person experiencing psychosis to know their experience best, resonates with the analytic approach of 'reversing' the transference in the first phase of treatment in psychosis (see Chap. 4).

Recall that the reversal of transference requires that the analyst become a student to the person experiencing psychosis. If we accept that voices and distressing beliefs (delusions) serve a purpose for the person experiencing psychosis, then it follows that they would have something to teach us as listeners and as clinicians. HVN has spontaneously discovered that it is imperative to begin by asking the person experiencing psychosis to explain how the voices and beliefs *work for them.*

This listening position, as Cindy's examples illustrate, is not a passive or silent one. Clearly, members of the HV group are quite active in expressing curiosity about the person's voices and beliefs. However, the questions are, ideally, not aimed at confirming or denying the truth, or existence, of the phenomena. Instead, with HVN, and with Cindy's examples in particular, the questions are 'real questions' in that the listener is inquiring from an authentic position of non-knowing and therefore from a position of 'wanting' to know.

In my assessment, there are two distinct phases in the HVN's approach to questioning which thus assert the possibility of 'challenge from within' to a person's voices and distressing beliefs. There is a first phase where the person experiencing psychosis engages in a process of explaining the content and logic of his or her voices and beliefs to other group members. The group member engages in explaining his or her beliefs in response to questions from other group members such as "how does that [belief] work?" or "how do you understand that [belief]?" or "how do they [voices] know that?" These are questions that privilege the perspective and knowledge of the person experiencing psychosis. If the group member has spent considerable time in the mental health system, these types of open and curious questions may surprise them because, in the mental health system, it is the norm for clinicians to probe the content of voices and delusions for 'risk factors' only, and to avoid asking about the meaning and context of voices and delusional beliefs. As social psychiatrist Dr. Marius Romme et al. (2009), a co-founder of the HVN, writes of "classical" psychiatry's aversion to listening, "[t]o listen to the person hearing voices was to collude with their delusion. The treatment was to ignore the voices and give the person medication to get rid of them" (Living with Voices, p. 73). Here Romme is referring to a period in psychiatry in the late 1980s when the HVN was founded. Sadly, the discipline of psychiatry, certainly within the U.S., continues to train its clinicians to ignore the meaning of psychotic phenomena and focus exclusively on the suppression of symptoms. Uncovering the meaning of the voices and delusional beliefs is not an end in itself but, instead, a first step towards challenging the beliefs and opening a path to discover the true source of a person's suffering.

There is a second phase in the HV group process where a member's belief system, or "framework", may begin to fail. The failing of the belief system, I suggest, is evidence of the power of the questioning and curiosity put forth between group members and, furthermore, marks the opportunity for the member to exit their delusion. In Cindy's earlier example, an HV group member transitions from beliefs that we might call delusional (e.g., voices/messages emanating from insects or through electrical wires) to a realization that his voices, beliefs, and distress correspond to a personal history of traumatic encounters. The member's journey from living within a fixed and isolating belief system to confronting the traumatic cause of his disturbance took time and perseverance by the member and also by others in the group who helped him uncover the meaning of his voices and beliefs.

As noted earlier, I believe that the HVN has 'spontaneously' discovered a mode of peer-driven treatment of voices and delusional beliefs. I am not entirely surprised by the similarities between the HVN approach and the analytic model that I have discussed in this book. The title of the introduction of this book is "The Psychotic as Guide", such that I take the psychotic's 'word' as true, as the place to begin the treatment, and as my compass point. My aim has been to reread Freud and Lacan through the lens provided by the experience of psychosis and, more importantly, to understand psychosis through listening to what people who experience psychosis say 'it' is. It has always been my conviction that we must begin with the experience of psychosis (as guide) in order to understand, live with, and/or exit the suffering of psychosis. Thus it does not surprise me that a peer-based approach, HVN, that listens to and follows the psychotic's experience has discovered very effective ways to intervene in psychosis and to effect change in the lives of people who experience psychosis. Nor does it surprise me that some of the most effective psychoanalytic methods with psychosis (e.g., ethical listening and questioning) look very similar to those discovered by the HVN.

In comparison to the HVN approach, there are also, generally speaking, two phases in the analytic approach to contesting the delusion with the aim of supporting the person experiencing psychosis in discovering the relationship between their voices, belief system (delusion), and traumatic history. In Chap. 4 of this book I discussed the challenge of how best to contest the certainty of delusion by way of (1) questioning and learning about the elements, structure, and purposes of delusional beliefs for the person experiencing psychosis and (2) by way of dream-work to evoke the person's subjective/traumatic history.

Delusion is often characterized by a knowledge or belief system that is totalizing and if, by mistake or misunderstanding, a clinician, peer, or family member attempts to contest the truth of the delusion or framework directly with consensual reality or 'reason', this attempt will often be met by the patient's shoring up of the belief system and/or a new elaboration of the belief system that in turn incorporates, or extinguishes, any 'doubt'. Similar to the effective approach of the HVN, the analyst may begin with supposing that delusion contains a knowledge that explains an experience that is true for the person experiencing psychosis. The delusion is viewed as a personal 'theory' or metaphor. The psychoanalytic view of delusion, as metaphor or theory, is similar to the HVN model where distressing beliefs are termed 'frameworks' and are understood as a way of explaining ('framing') underlying traumatic experiences.

Also, similarly to the HVN approach, the analyst adopts a position of curiosity by questioning the logic of delusion with questions similar to those used by peers in HV groups. The analyst adopts this position in order to learn more about the person's belief system and how the system works for the person. By questioning the delusion we can get a sense of the person's internal landscape including who is speaking through the voices, the content of the messages, what the person is being asked (or coerced) to do or not to do, and the various positions of suffering, power, or agency the person occupies in the scheme of his or her delusion.

The clinical example discussed in Chap. 6 provides a clear example of how the elements of the delusion are revealed by way of the analyst's curiosity and desire to know. As with the HVN approach, the analytic position can lead the person experiencing psychosis to a point where the logic of delusion reaches a limit or point of 'failure'. The patient arrived at a point in the treatment where the logic of his delusion resulted in a contradiction, or 'double-bind', where he was trapped between two untenable choices. For example, the patient stated: "The Supreme Beings say I *must* become a Nobel Laureate"; however, the patient also stated: "my mother and brother and I will be killed if I become a Nobel Laureate". I described this point in the treatment as an impasse and it was also at this point in the treatment where I asked the patient to speak about his dreams. Through his dream-work he recalled pieces of his subjective and traumatic history that, as I discussed, 'paralleled' certain moments and figures in his delusion, thus setting up a field of 'contestation' between the field of his subjective history and the field of his delusion. I hypothesized that the contestation itself, and the analyst's curiosity about the contestation, led the patient to raise a question about what he called the "truth of my delusion" (see Chap. 6, pp. 90–92 for elaboration of the logic of the treatment).

In both the HVN and the psychoanalytic approaches a rigid framework or delusion may be brought to a point of failure by the benevolent force of genuine curiosity and questioning. Furthermore, in both approaches, the 'point of failure' within the delusion brings forth the possibility of a new freedom for the person to confront the true source of their disturbance and suffering.

Returning to the interview

BF:

How do people respond to your stance of 'not knowing' and to your admission that they are the 'one who knows' about their own experience?

CMH:

They're not used to it. But it's disarming. And for so many people with unusual experiences, they have a history, a lot of times, of being told "you're wrong, you're wrong, you're wrong". And for somebody to say "You're right. I don't understand" can be really liberating for them. And then, what comes out sometimes is bigger and deeper than anything they've even had a conversation with themselves about.

BF:

Well, this seems to relate to what we've discussed in previous exchanges on the responsibility *for* versus responsibility *to* someone.

CMH:

Right. I can sit there and say: "I'm sure I know what's going on for this person." But that is not my job. That's not a success. It's for the person to come up with their answers and what makes sense to them. And then, they are part of their own rescue and they're taking responsibility and they're figuring out something that works for them. I'm not arrogant enough to think I know the answers for anyone else. My job is more about expanding possibilities.

[*Here Cindy provides an example of a change in frameworks from her own recovery*] When I was going to the Hearing Voices groups early on, I had this phenomenon of [hearing] a crying baby, and I came to find out there are many people who have this phenomenon of hearing a crying baby. I would search the cabinets in my house, I would search everywhere … I'd be looking for this crying baby. And somebody in the group said to me: "Oh, that's your inner child." It pissed me off, because it didn't sound like my inner child. I said: "What are you talking about? You know, I just want it to shut up." But I had to come to that place on my own, over time. Telling me "Oh, that's your inner child" was not helpful. What was helpful to me was when others asked me: "*When does the voice come? What does it come in relationship to?*"

And then I was like "Oh, that crying baby … how does it work in my life?" I realized that it was letting me know when I'm in a situation where I'm not being treated well.

BF:

That's what you discovered?

CMH:

Yeah, eventually. Because it got to the point where, not only did I hear it, I had an occasion where I saw it. And people were like "What was going on? Where were you?" And in having that conversation, in that moment I realized 'Oh, that does make sense'. But when someone said to me "Oh, that's your inner child", I'm like "Oh, you read some psychology book".

BF: But someone else asked you *when does it come*?

CMH:

Right. So like when it got to the point where I saw it, then people asked: "What? Wow. What was going on when you saw it?" And I got to talk about that circumstance, and that's when the pieces fell together for me.

BF:

So that was a whole new chunk of understanding, I guess, about that?

CMH:

Oh, it was huge. Because my attitude was like many people's attitudes are: "oh, the voice is the enemy" or "I just need to get rid of it". Or "it's tormenting me, leave me alone. How do I make it stop?" What happened instead was that I could see that the voice served a purpose. And it was actually a friend or like it was a positive. It [the voice] had a message and that I needed to hear. It was a huge turning point for me. Because instead of feeling plagued or whatever. I was like "okay, this is actually here to tell me I need to pay attention to something". A total shift in attitude.

BF:

Did that shift in attitude and perspective have any effect [on] the presence of the crying baby as a voice?

CMH:

Yeah, because I didn't need to have a crying baby anymore. You know?

Editorial note:

Here we have an example of how a voice or vision can change fundamentally or even stop. Uncovering and learning to navigate the underlying cause of, and purpose for, a voice can in turn make the voice unnecessary. The process of uncovering and learning to navigate the underlying traumatic cause of the voice begins with a willingness to listen to the voice.

CMH:

In the HVN training, sometimes I compare a voice to a toddler. A toddler wants your attention, a two-year-old wants your attention. You might be able to say to the toddler "In a bit. In a bit". And then what does the toddler do? Well, sometimes they get distracted or sometimes they get more provocative. If you're not careful, the kid climbs on top of the refrigerator and is pouring the Cheerios on the floor because you haven't gotten up to make him breakfast—you did not pay attention to him so he became more provocative.

The other metaphor is the one about 'your car is making a noise'. "Ah, maybe that noise will go away. Maybe it's just gravel around your break discs or something." But you know, maybe not. Or you go over a bump and the noise comes back. I can turn on the radio and that can be my strategy around the noise. And if the noise gets louder, I can turn up the radio. And then eventually what happens? The tire falls off or the axle breaks. This is more a metaphor around taking psychiatric drugs. You know, I can take more and more drugs so I don't hear the voices, or perhaps they're not so loud. Or I can just ignore them and they'll get bigger and more creative. And more provocative to get my attention.

So what I learned around the lesson with the crying baby was, when something starts to happen, look at it. Don't wait for it to get huge. Look at it. What is coming up for me now? What is it coming in relationship to? What do I need to look at? In other words, *go towards the experience instead of running away.*

Now, in taking this more curious approach, I still have what I call spiritual experiences but I don't have the big negative things. I might have a little negative thing and then I'm trying to *figure out why* it's coming up.

7.3 Conclusion: A Sympathy Rooted in a Shared Experience of Groundlessness

What do people with lived experience, and the HVN in particular, have to teach clinicians about how to listen to and work with psychosis?

Most importantly, the effectiveness of the HV approach speaks to the vital importance of the ethic of the listener, regardless of whether the listener is a clinician or person with lived experience of psychosis. In this chapter I have defined this ethical position as a position characterized, first and foremost, by curiosity and respect for the experience of psychosis. But where does this curiosity and respect issue from? Clearly, in listening to Cindy speak of her own experience and the experience of others we can grasp that the capacity for true respect issues from the facts of Cindy's personal experience and her understanding of psychosis.

One can be fearful of something that is radically unfamiliar—the unknown—and voices, visions, and distressing beliefs can be experienced by a given listener as something radically other and therefore as frightening. On the other hand, people with lived experience of psychosis who have found a way to recover from, and with, disturbing psychotic experiences are perhaps the ideal listener for a person who may just be beginning to find words for their inner experience. A main strength of the HV approach stems from the listener's personal experience of psychosis and, most importantly, the person's success with learning to 'treat' and live with the experience. When Cindy listens to someone else's experience of psychosis she is not frightened and therefore she is able to be curious. The 'lack of fear' and the presence of curiosity are key to the listener's ability to be present with someone experiencing psychosis.

Peer-to-peer interactions, as practised in the HV group model, are founded upon a 'common ground'. What constitutes the common ground? As noted, a *peer* is someone who has lived through an experience of psychosis and is thus familiar with the stakes, pressures, and disturbances of the experience of psychosis. A peer is in true sympathy with the other's experience. This is sympathy defined, not as pity for the other's misfortune, but rather as something more akin to an 'understanding' or 'common feeling' between people. The 'common ground' to which I refer is a bridge between subjects that issues from a knowledge of trauma and, paradoxically, from a knowledge of the inherent 'groundlessness' of subjective experience.

The HVN approach teaches clinicians what is required to enter into psychotic experience in order to be a useful guide to the psychotic subject in search of a way out of the destructive side of psychosis. The medical model certainly does not provide us with a language to understand how to access this common ground—or common 'groundlessness'. The orthodox Lacanian approach is also ill-equipped to help us in this respect.[4] An integration of the ethic of the HV approach and contemporary Lacanian approaches provides us with the best opportunity to bridge the gap between psychotic and 'non-psychotic' experience.

[4] I will further explore the limits of the orthodox Lacanian concept of transference, as well as the question of 'sympathy', in Chap. 9, "Bridging the Gap Between Psychotic and Non-Psychotic Experience".

References

Inter-Voice: The international hearing voices network. (2021). http://www.intervoiceonline.org

Romme, M., Escher, S., Dillon, J., & Corstens, D. (2009). *Living with voices: 50 stories of recovery*. PCCS, Ltd Books.

8

The Fear of Psychosis: Part II

This chapter will continue the exploration of the 'fear of psychosis'. We will again follow the lead of people who are in a unique position to discover new insights into the problem and function of fear. In a conversation with Annie Rogers, Ph.D., we will discuss how to contest the fear-driven 'poor prognoses' that are often given to people experiencing psychosis by mental health professionals. Dr. Rogers is an analyst, scholar, and a person with a lived experience of psychosis, thus her insights into the problem of fear are particularly nuanced and valuable. With Dr. Rogers, we will also discuss the importance of a 'fearless' clinician in her own analysis and recovery. From a more clinical perspective, Dr. Rogers offers important insights into the status of the 'Other of the address' in psychosis and we explore modifications to the transference that are necessary in order to work in collaboration with a person experiencing psychosis.

The latter section of this chapter will focus on the insights offered by Dr. Barri Belnap in her capacity as a psychiatrist and psychotherapist on an inpatient unit. The key terms that emerge from my discussion with Dr. Belnap are *dignity* and *respect*. Dr. Belnap discusses how to respond to psychotic speech in a way that maintains the patient's dignity and the

B. Fimiani, *Psychosis and Extreme States*, The Palgrave Lacan Series,
https://doi.org/10.1007/978-3-030-75440-2_8

dignity of what the person in psychosis has to say. Furthermore, Dr. Belnap discusses the problematic of how 'authority' is represented and exercised by clinical staff. As I have argued throughout this book, the psychotic has a particular insight into the unfoundedness of the Law and thus the credibility of authority is highly problematic in psychosis. Drawing upon her vast clinical experience, Dr. Belnap articulates the potential of a non-abusive representation of authority where both clinician and patient can have the freedom to express the ambivalent experience of authority itself.

As in the previous chapter, the interview transcript will be interspersed with "editorial notes" at pivotal moments in our discussion to elaborate on key conceptual points raised in the course of the interview.

8.1 Interview with Annie Rogers, Ph.D.

Dr. Rogers is an author, artist, psychoanalyst, university professor, and she has a history of lived experience of psychosis. Her experience of psychosis and clinical work are well documented in her numerous books on the topics of psychosis, psychoanalysis, art, and literature including *A Shining Affliction* (1995), *The Unsayable* (2006), and *Incandescent Alphabets* (2016). I first met Dr. Rogers in the early 2000s in Quebec City where we were both attending the yearly training seminars in psychoanalysis offered by GIFRIC. Dr. Rogers' input on the topic of 'fear' is particularly important due to her varied experience as a person who has lived through the experience of psychosis, as a scholar, and analyst in the Lacanian field.

When Dr. Rogers agreed to be interviewed for this book, I sent her the following questions to guide our discussion: As a person with lived experience of psychosis what is your experience of encountering fear in clinical settings? What do you think is missing from current mainstream clinical models that emphasize the 'management' of psychotic 'symptoms' versus approaches that view psychosis as a form of knowledge? What is your experience of encountering fear as a clinician with regard to other disciplines such as psychiatry, psychology, and medicine? Regarding the question of the 'address': What is the status of the Other of the address in psychosis? Is the Other destroyed or non-existent? Is the Other a perverse, abusive, and capricious entity? What position can the listener take (peer or analyst) to support the construction of a new address where a 'credible' Other can be built?

We began our discussion with a focus on her perspective regarding the presence of "fear" in clinical settings and she began by discussing how her encounter with a talented and curious—unfearful—clinician, an analyst, was instrumental in helping her live with, and work through, her own experiences of psychosis.

Dr. Annie Rogers (AR):

I think the gravest error that clinicians sometimes make is to assume that—because psychotic speech can sound disorganized—there's no address or no search for an address by the person experiencing psychosis.

However, having been in the experience of psychosis, and at the moments when I was most disorganized, people were indeed frightened. I know that people were frightened because, for example, my sister or very close friends would tell me that later. But in the moment, I didn't track that people were frightened because I was outside of the coordinates of space and time.

By the same token, when I first came to see the analyst that I wrote about in *A Shining Affliction*, whom I called Blumenfeld, I was in a pretty disorganized state. And I remember very distinctively going back to the house where I was staying afterwards and it was as if something had reset my compass in space and time. Enough so that when I went out for a walk with the family dog, I remember being absolutely astonished that I could keep track of where I was walking and I could walk back to the house.

I also remember, at the same time, being in no way impressed with this fellow I had just met. I observed his suit and his polished shoes; he appeared as a conventional analyst. But there was that other experience that gave me pause. "Who was this person who had affected me so strongly after meeting him once?"

For me the bottom line was that he communicated that *he was in no way frightened*—not by saying it—but by being fully present.

Editorial Note:

Dr. Rogers' reference to the 'resetting' of her compass is striking. The unique quality of her analyst's presence seems to have provided her with new 'coordinates'. Dr. Rogers' question "Who was this person that affected me…?" highlights the critical importance of the 'address' in the first meeting with someone experiencing psychosis. Her analyst, without fear and by being fully present as her listener, helped Dr. Rogers re-find her place in space and time. Blumenfeld, without saying much, somehow embodied courage, respect, and curiosity. Another way to characterize the effect of the analyst in this example is as someone who is able to be present in such a way that the person experiencing psychosis can use the analyst's presence in order to ground and orient themself.

AR:

I think the ways that people are frightened of psychosis are really quite evident. They were evident to me in my more lucid moments [when experiencing psychosis] and they're certainly very evident to me now. People want to pin down the diagnosis and make a correction, I suppose, in the most broad-minded sense, to bring the person [experiencing psychosis] more in line with a shared reality or just wanting to alter the symptom picture and call that treatment. And again, my experience is that, in terms of when I was young and it was clear that I was psychotic, the psychiatrist wanted to send me to the state hospital and I think that was their reaction of just plain fear: "What are we to do with this kid?"

Another time I thought "This is just sheer fear". There was one point where I didn't have very much money as an undergraduate and someone suggested to me that I could probably get disability money through social security and have a little bit of an income and a little more independence. And I thought "Well, why not?" So I went to check this out and see what was possible. The interview itself was very telling to me because the interviewer couldn't credit in any way that I could be in college, let alone be doing extraordinarily well in college because it didn't fit his picture of what someone in psychosis looks like. They wanted to send me to a series of skills-building classes as a condition for being in this programme. And, basically, he told me that I shouldn't have very high aspirations for my future. I remember it so clearly, Bret. I looked him in the eye and I said "If this is what you're telling me and offering me, I don't want this benefit. I don't want anything to do with it", and I got up and I walked out. And I am forever grateful when I look back on it that that was exactly my choice. Because again, I know people who are now in middle age and who, when they were young, identified to the position of psychosis, identified to that position and took in other people's fears and messages about it and then lived that.

Editorial Note:

Dr. Rogers expands further on how she was able to resist negative messages and poor prognoses suggested to her by professionals in the mental health system.

AR:

When I think about my own experience, in a way my mother was a protective force in my young life because she was largely in denial of what I was living through, in so far as she could grasp it at all. And in a curious kind of way it served me well. For example, when I was a junior in high school and I was not getting any better after seven months in a hospital, the psychiatrist suggested that I be transferred to the state hospital within the city. And my mother basically stepped in and said: "No way, she's coming home; she's going back to school."

So, I came home, on all these antipsychotic medications, and I went back to my really quite wonderful high school. I came off the medications secretly as soon as I could, and I struggled terribly through the end of that year, and the entire following summer actually; it was like a living nightmare. But then somehow in my last year in high school, I surfaced into this period of lucidity that I didn't experience again until I was almost in my mid-thirties. And it, the lucidity, allowed me to kind of live into my mother's belief that "Of course she'll go back to high school, she'll finish high school, everything will be well". But I think there was a promise of 'going back to school' as a possibility that I didn't want to turn my back on. And that stood me in very good stead when indeed I did go through crisis after crisis and hospitalization after hospitalization.

Editorial Note:

It is noteworthy that both Cindy Marty Hadge, in her interview in Chap. 7, and Dr. Rogers, in this chapter, underscore the importance of a person in their lives who addressed them in a specifically optimistic way while they were in crisis or struggling. For Cindy, her supervisor at the

Western Mass Recovery Learning Community reminded Cindy of her teaching responsibilities, which in turn compelled Cindy to conclude her hospitalization and return to her work. For Dr. Rogers, it was her mother who insisted, however seemingly far-fetched at the time, that she could indeed return to school and succeed. Furthermore, in Chap. 9, I will discuss the work of Françoise Davoine and Jean-Max Gaudilliere and their case study of "Gilda", who, in a time of lucidity and separation from her madness, reminded her analyst: "You told me, '*yes, it is possible to get out of madness*'." Cindy, Dr. Rogers, and Gilda all encountered someone (employer, mother, analyst) who believed that psychosis, as pure illness, was not destiny.

Return to interview

Now, when I meet young people who have been in psychosis or who are quite frankly in psychosis, I ask them what they've been told about their diagnosis and their future and I challenge it. I just directly challenge it. And I encourage them to consider their future and to consider who they would like to become, what really interests them, what it will take for them to hold onto those things. I especially ask them what are the gifts of their own mind that they can experience through this period of crisis. And hopefully it makes some difference. It's not always a psychoanalytic kind of intervention. It's just an intervention coming from someone who has lived through it.

I think of someone like my friend John Devlin. He is a psychotic artist that I've connected with in Canada, a man around the same age as me, and he also received all of these awful messages regarding his prognosis. He didn't have access to psychoanalysis. He lives in a group-home but he's made art for four decades and he knows how to navigate his experience as a kind of gift of psychosis. And right now he's really concerned with the question of *who will remember him, where will his artwork be archived, who can learn from it?* Well, that's a much bigger question than just *how do I get through life from day to day*?

I have reached out to people to see if I can find a place that will archive his work and some of the articles about him, and make a kind of lasting place for him. Because at this stage in our lives, as for many people in their sixties, the question of legacy comes up. It's a human question. What will become of what I've tried to give to the world after I'm gone?

And at the other end of the spectrum, being in your twenties and being told by professionals that you will have no life, no future, that you will be on medication indefinitely, in and out of the hospital, no chance to have family—these kinds of messages set the bar very low. Well, in terms of John's legacy, I want to set the bar high.

Bret Fimiani (BF):

And what kind of response do you get from young people when you challenge what they have been told about their prognosis? How do people respond to your challenge?

AR:

Well, definitely with relief, with gladness. But the way forward for them may not be all that clear at the beginning. Someone may have set their sights on a particular academic degree and it's going to take years longer to get there. Or, they may have set their sights on wanting to travel to a part of the world and [...] work there. And that, as a possibility, given the severity of the crisis, [...] may not be able to happen for a while. So their own path is not yet clear to them and yet there's a real sense of relief and hope. And even when they have to call into question some of the things that they think [...] they know there is still a space for their own knowing.

BF:

Is there anything more you could say about how you knew that your analyst was not afraid? It could be helpful for clinicians to hear, from your point of view, how you knew that it was safe there in his office and that you were welcome to speak about your experience of psychosis.

AR:

It was partly the quality of his silence. He was very, very present and persistent without being a nudge, very persistent. I remember [psychiatrist and psychoanalyst] Charles Turk talking about following a young patient from room to room in this [hospital] ward of rooms, just trying to have a conversation. And while it wasn't quite that with my analyst, I remember at the end of the session he asked if I would like to see him again the next day. And that was a very big signal to me that he was not afraid. But, actually, I don't know how I knew that because even in retrospect, I know that I was in pretty bad shape in terms of being able to navigate the world at that time. For example, I was staying with the family of a former college professor for a time, and the woman of the house asked me if I would draw a picture of what was planted in the backyard because she wanted to plant some other things. My picture of the backyard didn't resemble the backyard at all. And I remember trying to walk up a flight of stairs and the flight of stairs would not hold still enough for me to know how to climb it. So, I was not in good shape.

I don't know how I knew [...] about this analyst's lack of fear—but I did. And I think in terms of being a clinician, that quality of a presence and real interest in knowing what's going on for that person in psychosis, that quality just matters enormously.

BF:

Real interest. Well, the word *persistent* really stands out to me as a manifestation of desire itself somehow, or of the *desire of the analyst* perhaps.

AR:

I think this is absolutely right.

Editorial Note:

Blumenfeld's position as a listener recalls Françoise Davoine and Jean-Max Gaudilliere's application of the concept of "zone of non-existence",[1] which is a zone that both patient and clinician must enter into in order to find a way out of psychosis—the analyst cannot hide from or avoid this zone. I will explore and develop the relationship between transference and the concept of "zones of non-existence" in depth in Chap. 9. However, a brief reference to the importance of a common "zone" that draws in both patient and analyst will be useful here to illuminate how important Dr. Rogers' observations about Blumenfeld and Charles Turk are in fact.

Blumenfeld offers a place and time to speak and he must have recognized or 'known' that psychotic speech has meaning. Dr. Rogers' passing reference to psychiatrist and psychoanalyst Charles Turk is instructive as well. The anecdote involving Turk sheds light on the importance of persistence on the side of the analyst. As Dr. Rogers notes, Turk followed "a

---

[1] Françoise Davoine and Jean-Max Gaudilliere adopted the concept of "zone of non-existence" from psychoanalyst Gaetano Benedetti (1920–2013). See Françoise Davoine and Jean-Max Gaudilliere's discussion and application of this concept in *History Beyond Trauma* (2004) and in *Madness and the Social Link* (2021).

young patient from room to room in this [hospital] ward of rooms, just trying to have a conversation". It is clear, by the statement "following from room to room" that Turk also believed that psychotic speech is meaningful and purposeful and that "conversation" was possible. A belief or 'conviction' that a conversation was possible was offered to a patient. Such an offering is not so common on most hospital wards. The responsibility is then on the side of the person in psychosis to 'accept' such an offer, and this is precisely what Dr. Rogers chose to do when receiving an offer from Blumenfeld to speak of her experience. The address, 'structured as it is by the relation of subject to the O/other, is forged when both analyst and patient enter into an agreement to truly listen to what the psychotic has to say. In other words, the address is 'co-created' between the listener and the person experiencing psychosis.

In what follows Dr. Rogers begins to discuss the problem of the "address" in psychosis. Who, what Other, is the person experiencing psychosis speaking to, and when? What position can the clinician adopt in order to receive what the person experiencing psychosis has to say?

BF:

The question of the address, and how the address differs in psychosis versus neurosis, interests me.

AR:

It interests me, too, because I think the address can be all over the map in psychosis. I mean, there's not just one 'other of the address'. There are times when the person in psychosis is not primarily addressing the person in the room. They are taking into account, *in* their address, other entities or forces or people who are *listening in* and even giving them their words to say.

BF:

You talk about *the multiple* a lot, especially in Chap. 7 of your recent book [*Incandescent Alphabets*].

AR:

Yes. There are times when the psychotic person in the room is really trying to say something very compelling about their experience, and it's being read [by the listener] as a manifestation of psychosis itself. And then that's it. That's the end of it. The psychotic person recognizes that there's no response, there's no question, there's no interest, there's no true inquiry, there's simply no there there in *that* other to even reach toward.

BF:

This sounds like, for example, when a listener is just trying to identify the diagnosis per the DSM for example. It is not in any way considered that the person experiencing psychosis has something to say that is meaningful.

AR:

For example, recently I was asked to do a consultation around a patient who's potentially psychotic. And the person asking for the referral wrote back to me and said: "Well, this patient doesn't understand that this is a 'delusion' so, what's the sense of doing a consultation?" And I wrote back to the clinician and basically said: "If you want to make a space for this person to speak, it's worth doing the consultation. Of course they don't understand their own thinking as a delusion. *From their point of view, it's not.*"

And again, within the address, I realize sometimes the person in psychosis really does believe they know something that other people don't have any access to. And they may be unwilling to speak. This becomes doubly hard if what they have to say is [...] met with absolute incredulity [by the listener]. It may also be difficult to speak because the person is so convinced and so certain of what they know, that, in a sense, they lose track of the fact that others don't inhabit the same world.

I remember very clearly as an adolescent, there was an upstairs neighbour who was a librarian whom I grew very close to. And she had tin foil all over the ceiling of her apartment. And she thought that aliens were listening in and observing her all the time. And she did not speak of her experience in the world because she was a librarian and there's no way she could have kept her job if she revealed her experience. But she believed it so strongly that it affected everything she said and did.

And she recognized something in me that allowed her to tell me exactly why her apartment was constructed in the way that it was. And I remember such relief that that could be spoken. I didn't reciprocate, but I remember such profound relief that it could be spoken.

BF:

How old were you at that time?

AR:

Maybe 17.

BF:

Okay, so you were having your own experiences?

AR:

Yes.

BF:

So, that was very welcoming of you, providing an 'address' or a credible other, indirectly, perhaps?

AR:

Yes, but again, she had to have a pretty clear sense of the *other of her address* to be able to know who not to speak to and who to speak to. Whereas there are other times in psychosis where I think, in more disorganized states, when the psychotic person, as they're speaking, they are not really keeping track of other people's responses because they can't. And in that sense, there's something about the other of the address that is just *gone.*

BF:

In those moments of disorganization?

AR:

Yes. And then, your question of 'how do you build a credible other?' From those kinds of moments, I think it's extremely delicate and elusive and difficult to inhabit. But again, the person who's in psychosis recognizes such a person.

BF:

Would your neighbour who experienced psychosis have known that you were having somewhat similar experiences?

AR:

She would have known, for instance, Bret that I had just come out of a long psychiatric hospitalization at age 17. Because we lived in an apartment building where there were just six families. And that was a time in American history when neighbours knew neighbours and basically what was going on with each other. And that was a time when I really couldn't navigate walking the two blocks I needed to get to my high school. I just could not manage time and space in that way. And she would drive me to school in the morning on her way to the library. She dropped me off at school because we didn't have a family car. And so, I mean, she did know.

BF:

Okay. So, that's what she knew. She knew that *you knew* something of the experience perhaps? She opened up to you about her psychotic experience and she spoke to you about something that she could not speak about to most others.

AR:

Yes.

Editorial Note:

In what follows Dr. Rogers elaborates on variations of the 'Other of the address' where the Other could be "gone", and "enigma", "controlling and omniscient", and finally the Other as a "far horizon".

AR:

It's interesting. I think there are moments when the other of the address is gone because there's such chaos. And I think there are moments when the other is a place of profound enigma that's really deeply unsettling. And then, I think there's a place where there's been, in my view, a building of an incandescent alphabet, a new code, a new order, a new something, that would answer that enigma. And then the other becomes something else—sometimes controlling, sometimes omniscient and controlling, sometimes simply a force to contend with, but that Other also gives the person in psychosis a place and a purpose. And then, I think there's also the experience of the other as, how do I describe this, a far horizon. I think of it as trying to speak against a language divide. If you've ever had an experience of being in a foreign country where you are a visitor and you didn't know the language and you had to figure out through gestures and signs how to say something to other people—that's the other as a far horizon—where it just seems inconceivable to be able to find the right words to reach that horizon.

I've been deeply interested in the process of coming back from 'psychosis-as-crisis' gradually into a different experience of *psychosis as a much more stable position* where the other of the address changes and becomes something else. I'm recalling my own experience of not hearing errors in language in my own speech, and then at one point beginning to hear them. I remember suddenly seeing that I was taking what was metaphor too literally, or hearing that I'd just replaced a word with another inappropriate word, simply because I just couldn't find words; the words would disappear. But then, I realized: "Oh, the words were disappearing." That's not the same thing as being in complete chaos. It's in fact far more frightening an experience because then the other is truly this far horizon. How could you arrive into it to speak?

BF:

A question about the "Other as far horizon" metaphor: So, a "horizon", by definition, is a 'place' that one never reaches, yes? In the general sense I think of a 'horizon' as the *appearance* of a limit or place that one cannot reach.

AR:

Well, [...] that's one of the profound places of convergence in neurosis and in psychosis that can happen at some point. The neurotic really understands what is lacking in language, and realizes that no matter how often they try to say something that's truly almost memorable, but not memorable, or something of an experience of real trauma that you don't have the words to say—you *can only go so far*. And the other of your own address is always elusive. There's always more to say. And in psychosis, I think that initial experience of the other as a far horizon is far more hopeless. Yet I have learned that a seeming impossibility of speaking can become an approximation, *a way of saying that does not attempt to say everything*. And for the psychotic to understand that you can't say everything of your experience is huge. It actually allows one to speak.

BF:

Returning to your comment about a 'point of convergence' in neurosis and psychosis and with regard to the experience of psychoanalysis: Do you think that there's a point in the analytic experience—meaning the work of the unconscious—where the psychotic and non-psychotic are in the same position with regard to an Other, for example? An other that is at the horizon—that place one cannot go *to, or into*?

AR:

Yes. For example, I interviewed John Devlin. He is structurally psychotic and not in crisis, but quite stabilized between his practice of art and his low-dose medications. And the result is that when you speak to him, you can create a very lucid space. And he and I both spoke about our experiences. And there are times when he just laughed because he knew that what he was trying to put into words was something that was just impossible to put into words. Yeah. He was able to accept that there's a certain level of the *absence of the other* and he is simply unable to say certain things. I think, too, of a man I have known as an analysand for some time, and how he now can laugh at his own slips, at his nonsense, which speaks without him. He is neurotic, but at times his own speech becomes a far horizon.

BF:

This makes me think again about the question of fear. I was at a lecture once where Willy Apollon said: "It's not a question of *why* someone is psychotic but, more to the point, why are we not all psychotic?" Which I think suggests there's a common place that we're all coming from, experientially, and in terms of subject formation. What do you think?

AR:

Yes, I think that is a profound question posed by Willy Apollon. We have more in common in our origins than one might imagine. None of us recall early childhood experience, especially the experience of the other as voice, as enigma and whim, and the child's sense that the *jouissance of the other* can be used in an all-powerful way for or against her. This early experience of language itself as enigmatic and all the bodily disorganization that goes with that returns in psychosis. Indeed, why not to all of us?

8.1.1 Conceptual Interlude: "The Other as Far Horizon"

Dr. Rogers gives us a new language to try to grasp how different versions of the 'other of the address' appear and function in psychosis. There are different 'moments' in the experience of psychosis when the other of the address takes different forms and assumes different purposes for the person experiencing psychosis.

In moments of profound disorganization and "chaos" the other is "gone", perhaps non-existent, or destroyed. There are other moments when the other is multiple in that the person in psychosis is not addressing the 'person in the room' but is, in Dr. Rogers' terms, "taking into account, in their address, other [perhaps many] entities or forces or people who are listening in and even giving them words to say".

There are moments when the other, perhaps in a more consolidated form, is a "place" of "profound enigma". As Dr. Rogers powerfully states, the other as enigma is "deeply unsettling". The enigmatic and unsettling other then calls for a response from the subject—an answer? The call to respond to the other's enigma sets the psychotic subject to work to find a way to solve the puzzle imposed by the other. The 'work' may take the form of "becoming a Nobel Laureate", as my clinical discussion in Chap. 6 illustrated or, as in Dr. Rogers' example, the creation of "incandescent alphabets".[2]

Finally we have the "other as a far horizon". How does the other as "profound enigma" differ from the other as "far horizon?" A key difference appears to be that the other as far horizon represents a limit whereas the other as enigma, being as it is linked to capricious demands, is in practice unlimited or, in Lacanian terms, 'unbarred'. And, in Dr. Rogers' explanation, the other as far horizon evokes an experience of the limit of language itself and the impossibility of 'saying it all'. As she notes, "[f]or the psychotic to understand that you *cannot say everything* of your experience is huge". Does the confrontation with the other as far horizon open up the possibility of symbolic castration for the psychotic?

8.1.2 The Relevance of Lacan and the Limits of the Orthodox Lacanian Concept of the Analyst's Position with Psychosis

AR:

With psychosis, versus neurosis, the problem is *not* to be able to speak freely. Rather, in psychosis, the problem is to be able to make language work, to be able to, as you said, construct an address that works. And I think it calls for the person on the other side of that, the analyst or whoever it might be, *to be exquisitely aware of how little they in fact know*

[2] See Dr. Rogers' most recent book: *Incandescent Alphabets: Psychosis and the Enigma of Language* (2016).

of this experience while trusting that there are things they can know about the experience. It is an experience of being shattered, of trauma, of waking up and not knowing where you are or how language works—these are experiences of terror. These are human experiences. And in that sense, there is a way to come forward and to meet a person who is really terrified of what's unfolding.

And I think it's vital, this wanting to know more of that person's experience. Because the person who is in psychosis has no reason whatsoever to trust that person to receive what they have to say, to receive it as knowledge, or to receive it as knowledge that should be taken seriously. So, it's a lot of work to get there. And then language itself may not be working in so many ways, such that it is literally difficult to speak. Listening on the other side of that, you have to really believe that there is a subject that's in disarray, but it's trying to say something. And I think that to really accompany that 'saying' you have to be as inventive as you can possibly be. I mean, in that sense, there's no orthodoxy that could tell you how to act, or say how *to be* from moment to moment. The intervention is judged by its effects. It's the same thing with someone in psychosis: you invent, moment by moment.

And if the challenge with the neurotic is to get them to be interested in the idea that there's something other than their version of reality and the endlessly repeating loops of torment that they put themselves and other people through, then the challenge with psychosis is to be able to get them to see some crack in the very premises of the delusion so they can become genuinely curious about what this experience is, and what they've built it out of, and how to begin to dismantle some little pieces of it to open up a new direction in some way. And so it doesn't mean just being empathic and listening, and finding out more and more and more about delusion; although that's very important, it's not the limit of it.

BF:

On the question of Lacan's contribution in particular, could you speak to what is most relevant and important to you about Lacan's work with regard to understanding psychosis?

AR:

A good bit of Lacan from his *Seminar III*, and some pieces of *Seminar XXIII* are important to me. From *Seminar XXIII*, remember that James

Joyce did not have a crisis of madness. He did not end up in and out of asylums and hospitals being treated for madness. Joyce built a life structurally in psychosis. And that I think is just huge. If you really take that in what you've got to acknowledge the question 'How is it possible for someone to do this?'

The other thing that Lacan talks about in *Seminar XXIII* that I find incredibly compelling is his idea of the "open ego". The ego in *Seminar III* reduplicates itself. But in *Seminar XXIII* the 'open' ego refers to the person who's not attached to particular emotions or particular ideas—the open ego doesn't get involved at that level of attachment because things shift around almost too quickly for that. For me this open ego offers gifts of being able to see things in fresh ways over and over again. I think psychosis contains important knowledges for our time. This knowledge involves learning from an experience of crisis, a trajectory *through and beyond* psychosis (as it is triggered again and again), or psychosis *as a lived experience* without undergoing a crisis of madness.

What I find incredibly helpful in that early seminar, *Seminar III*, is thinking about the idea that it's not hallucination per se that defines psychosis, but rather the *effects* of hallucination. It's not necessarily a voice; it could just be an experience. But it's an experience in which there's an address from an Other that is made specifically to the subject and that places him or her in a very specific position that there's no escape from, no escape from that experience of the Other that usually repeats. And the effect of that is the building of all kinds of defences, including delusions to live in that situation in psychosis. I find that incredibly helpful as a way of thinking.

The analysts of GIFRIC have been helpful in giving us the idea that 'Yes, you can work with dreams with people in psychosis, but the first dreams will be reiterations of the universe that they've constructed in delusion'. And it's only when there's something else, some other signifier, some other question that comes to bear an Other scene, that there is then a crack into a different logic outside of the suppositions that are made in delusion. And again, that was just really profound learning for me.

BF:

You said psychosis is not defined by hallucinations, but by the *effect* of hallucinations, and that Lacan articulates this distinction in *Seminar III*. Can you elaborate on this idea?

AR:

Yes, in *Seminar III* Lacan talks about a young woman who encounters a man in her apartment building and she doesn't understand what the man says to her regarding a potential sexual liaison he had within the building. It confuses her—that terrain of sexuality. And so she misinterprets what he has to say and interprets his intent in a paranoid way. That's one piece where it's not a voice. It's an actual experience with an individual in reality.

But then I think about Schreber as well. The little men who inhabit his body, all over his body, he always puts them in quotes. Schreber even describes the little men at one point; he says "I can see them vividly in my mind's eye". He knows that they're not of the same status as, let's say, the "attendants" that are coming and going. They are far more intimate and far more destructive, and they have far more power over him. So it's not just that he experiences these things visually or verbally or in his body. The effect of it [the experience of sensations invading the body] is to create an experience of the Other that has taken over his body and ultimately, of course, the effect is to cause Schreber to build a delusion such that 'God is someone who wants to turn him into a woman so that God can impregnate him and there can be a new birth to humanity'. So it goes that far. But the delusion is the effect of an experience, not the experience per se.

BF:

That is the effect of, can we say, "the break-in of the Voice" (as Willy Apollon uses the term) or the effect of the *emergence* of voice? I think we're getting into something very difficult and important, which is the question of causality. Some clinicians find the question of causality or the 'origin' of psychosis vital and some do not. For example, psychiatrist Barri Belnap doesn't think causality is key, but rather she focuses only on what the person experiencing psychosis is saying and constructing, which are precisely the 'effects'—when the person experiencing psychosis (chaos, permeability, terror) speaks, we are hearing that particular subject's 'response' to the experience. There are voices, there are experiences of invasion, and then there's the effects of that and the response to that through speech, psychotic speech.

AR:

Exactly.

BF:

And this may come in the form of an elaborate delusion. This is not unlike how analyst Lucie Cantin would frame it: "The delusion is a theory of an experience."

AR:

Yes, and that theory can seal the psychotic into a closed universe in which the same terrifying experiences repeat and repeat. Stijn Vanheule actually talks about the idea of resistance to this repetition and enclosure. He talks about autonyms in speech that Lacan first identified as coming from the Other. Vanheule noticed that these autonyms increasingly become adopted into the discourse of the psychotic. They become owned by the psychotic and used in relation to an Other that's destructive and has completely taken over the psychotic person's life. There's a little edge of resistance taken up in the mission itself. Because to really take up the mission, you've got to appoint yourself in some way as an agent. I find that really potentially very powerful in terms of treatment.

For me, the 'origin' question has to do with contingency—what is associated with this rupture when it first happened? What was at stake in the rupture and then what was left so blown open that that the voice(s) came in over and over again until the person finally built a structure of response to it that they could live with? So it's less about cause or even origins and more a question of contingency. What was that experience? It cannot be remembered, but sometimes it can be constructed.

8.1.3 Conclusion: "What Was That Experience?"

What was that experience *of* rupture? Dr. Rogers teaches us that the phenomenology of psychosis—voices and delusions—are responses to an experience of rupture. As she asks, "what was left so blown open that the voices came in over and over…?" What happened to the subject, to the person, such that the person had to build a particular type of structure to make sense of the experience? The experience of rupture is common to all subjects, not only for psychotic subjects. Therefore I am not suggesting that rupture or 'trauma' is the source, or cause, of psychosis. Rather the question is how does *a* subject respond to an experience of rupture?

There is a place and moment that is characterized by the rupture itself and in psychosis the voice rushes in to fill the void left by the rupture. 'Voices' can be single words, random sounds, and brief phrases carrying special messages. Sometimes messages arrive to the subject without reliance upon an audible voice. Voices and messages can be fragmentary and free from any overarching narrative or explanation. The building of a structure—a "framework" or "delusion"—constitutes a phase of the psychotic experience where the subject, out of necessity, creates a separate world where the messages take on a clear purpose and typically afford the subject a new sense of agency as well. The agency of the subject of psychosis, or what Dr. Rogers calls a "little edge of resistance", is an effect of what Dr. Rogers refers to as the "mission".[3] The mission is a facet of the 'framework' or delusion exemplified in Chap. 6 of this book where the person under discussion is 'chosen' by the "Supreme Beings" to "be a Nobel Laureate".

Dr. Rogers asks what was at stake in the rupture. This is a key question that should be kept in mind when guiding any treatment of psychosis. In the course of treatment, knowledge of the rupture emerges in connection with remembered encounters with a particular force, or some 'other', that threatens the subject and against which the subject has no symbolic resources to protect herself or to make sense of the experience of the rupture.

[3] "Mission" is a term used by Apollon et al. (2002) of GIFRIC to describe how the psychotic person may be 'elected' or 'chosen' to "repair a defect in the universe". See Chap. 6 of this book for a full discussion of how being "elected" to such a role or function affords the psychotic subject agency and may indeed constitute a form of "resistance", as Dr. Rogers suggests earlier.

8.2 Interview with Barri Belnap, MD: Psychiatry and the "Dignity" of Psychosis

Prior to my conversation with Dr. Belnap I sent her the following questions to guide our discussion. What is your experience of working with people who experience psychosis in a hospital setting? What is your experience of encountering fear as a clinician? As someone who is trained analytically and medically how do you view the disconnect between the medical (i.e., bio-psychiatric) model and an analytic approach to listening to psychosis? You have written on the topic of "patient authority and treatment resistance". How do you maintain the conditions for 'patient authority' in the hospital setting where the medical model often approaches people experiencing psychosis as passive recipients of treatment?

I first became aware of Dr. Belnap's work when reading a chapter in *The Austen Riggs Reader* titled "What Is Psychodynamic Psychopharmacology? An Approach to Pharmacologic Treatment Resistance" (2011) by Dr. Belnap and Dr. Mintz. At the time I was working in an 'integrated primary care clinic' and I was struggling to find a way to initiate a psychoanalytically informed discussion with medical providers about 'treatment resistance' to antipsychotic and mood-stabilizing drugs. As both a psychoanalyst and a psychiatrist, Dr. Belnap is very well positioned to speak about the impasses reached by bio-psychiatry with regard to psychosis and illuminate how, in her view, psychoanalytic listening can be brought to bear in a medical setting. Dr. Belnap also has very important insights into how the fear of psychosis can be overcome by adopting a listening position that affords people experiencing psychosis, and their messages, dignity and importance.

With regard to the topic of the 'fear of psychosis' in clinical settings, Dr. Belnap began by discussing her experience working in a psychiatric hospital unit and witnessing an interaction where a mental health worker skilfully engaged a person experiencing a crisis. The clinical anecdote that Dr. Belnap refers to in our conversation is an example that she described in detail in her paper titled "Security: a process of working together when things go bad". I will quote her paper at length in order give a proper context to the interview material that follows.

In her paper, Dr. Belnap provides an example of how a clinician can act from a place of curiosity and compassion, rather than from fear. In particular, Dr. Belnap explores how "treating someone with dignity" can create a sense of trust and "security". The assertion that 'treating someone with dignity may create trust' may not, at first glance, appear to be a novel insight. However, the power of Dr. Belnap's observation becomes evident once one recognizes the inherent challenge, due to social stigma and misunderstanding, of attributing 'dignity' to psychotic experiences and psychotic speech. The Latin root of the word dignity is *dignus*, which means 'worth' or the quality of 'being worthy'. The attribution of dignity to psychotic experiences implies that the listener attributes worth to what the person in psychosis is saying.

Dr. Belnap draws a contrast between 'treating psychotic speech with dignity' and the more common approach to perceived danger in a hospital setting, which is to approach the experience of psychosis exclusively as a brain disease, thus rendering psychotic speech meaningless. It is certain that providers who follow the medical model attribute worth and dignity to their patients. I would never suggest otherwise. However, I am being more specific here as I am distinguishing between attributing worth to the person and worth to what a person 'says'. Another way of formulating the question of worth is to reassert the claim that the analytic model supposes that there is a 'subject' (a 'knowing' subject) of psychotic speech whereas the medical model does not. From a purely bio-psychiatric perspective, voices, visions, and distressing beliefs are understood as malfunctions of the brain and are treated as such. The act of listening for the subject in psychotic speech by definition 'dignifies' the person *and* their messages.

The following is an excerpt from Dr. Belnap's unpublished paper (2015) "Security: a process of working together when things go bad".

> I walked onto the unit of the locked psychiatric ward. I could hear screaming and banging of doors. Strangely the unit was otherwise calm and quiet. The other teenagers were going about their activities and chatting.

A woman was standing next to a boy who towered over her. His face was pressed against the window of the door that he was pounding on with his fists. He was yelling and threatened "*them*" if they tried anything. He wouldn't stand for it he said. He gave the impression of someone ferocious—someone who would not be toyed with. If anyone wanted to harm him he was making it known [that] he would fight *them* this time.

A tall male nurse stood quietly to the side. The young woman was talking to the 16-year-old boy with great lightness and warmth.

I heard her say: "I know that you know I am standing here beside you … and I know that while you are very upset at them, you don't want to hurt me.

I live in multiple worlds too and I see that you are very angry at people I cannot see, but I am here and I know you don't want to hurt me.

Would you like to come with me to the other room and tell me whatever you wish about the people you are talking to[?] We could play cards as we talk if you like."

The young man looked protectively at the small woman, turned back to the door and after a last few angry words and gestures he followed her into the game room … the two of them looking like friends comfortable in the familiarity of each other's presence.

Later after I read about this boy in the chart, I realized how obviously appropriate his behavior was and how important. This was a boy who was bullied and abandoned. He had been the object of racial prejudice, a witness to violence towards his mother and someone whom life had shown that cruelty was possible and probable at times. He had been unable to speak for himself or [a]ffect these violent others who intended and delivered harm to himself and his mother.

He was, in relation to that world, doing things differently. In this world—here on the unit of a psychiatric ward—he was speaking and showing himself capable of protecting himself and others by yelling at "them" and saying he would not stand for it again, not this time.

Whereas at times before, no one came to his aid, not even himself, he was now showing himself and the world the kind of boy he was or perhaps the kind of man he would consider trying to be. He was re-visioning the future and building on a past that knew the way inhumanity is always a presence in the world.

I asked the young woman how she did it—what was her method? who taught her?

She said simply, "I try to do my best to treat everyone with dignity."

Dignity. She did not try to offer care, or empathy, or advice or instruction. No support was necessary.

She simply treated him with dignity. From a place of dignity he could join her in playing a game. Being met with dignity, it seems, was enough for safety to be created—a sense of safety from which he could choose to leave behind the aspects of his past that had for a moment been reminding him of how bad things could be.

Dignity.

The intuition of the young woman on the unit comes to mind. His living in many worlds reminded her that she too lived in many worlds. Their bond was based on a mutual discovery and on her listening well for the voice she did not necessarily expect to hear. Dr. Jill Stauffer, in her book *Ethical Loneliness: The Injustice of Not Being Heard* (2015), suggests instances of "not hearing a person's suffering communicated in his or her own terms is unethical because not doing so affects the capacity for trust in the world." Her regarding him with dignity seemed to restore trust in the world as being large enough to include him and her and possibilities neither had thought of yet.

Editorial Note:

The mental health worker's statement "I know that while you are very upset at them, you don't want to hurt me" is important. The mental health worker 'knows' something, but how does she know it? As Dr. Belnap explains, the mental health worker's personal and cultural history affords her an intimate understanding of "living in multiple worlds" and the isolation, fear, and misunderstanding that unusual and extreme experiences can evoke in the self and in others. The mental health worker is making a wager of sorts. She cannot know with certainty what the patient 'wants', or doesn't want; however, she offers the patient a chance to 'play' (cards) and to speak in a different space and in a different way. The mental health worker spoke from a place of mutual understanding of an experience of alienation and of being misunderstood. As Dr. Belnap notes, "[t]heir bond was based on a mutual discovery". In the moments following the intervention the patient had a choice to engage the mental health worker in a way that could prevent a repetition of 'things going badly'.

BF:

The mental health worker said: "I treat him with dignity." Can you speak about what you think was key in the success of her intervention?

BB:

Well I think it was many steps. She had a link with the patient. She assumed that he was speaking in a meaningful way. She imagined it to work for him and found its meaningfulness. She spoke to all the parts of him at the same time, not just the one that represented her fear. So she said: "I know you don't want to hurt me." She also offered him another place to go and to do something else, to 'play, to play a game so that this reality could exist, and they could also have another space. So she reminded him that they have many spaces that they existed in together that she validated, and could speak about and respect. She also said that she too had personal experiences that could link her to what he was talking about.

Because of her cultural experience she had no trouble sharing parts of herself with the patient—she was not afraid or ashamed. She knows a lot about how many things can be true at the same time and about how an experience that is meaningful to you may not be meaningful or recognizable to other people. She [mental health worker] shows that you can be in a difficult moment and read that moment from various aspects of your cultural experience and from your history. She didn't have to act like "none of us know about that". I think she also did the imaginative work to see how this person is like herself and wasn't ashamed to see and share her own conflictual experiences.

Furthermore, I think she substitutes respect for what other people would argue is safety. She didn't talk about safety at all. She offered respect. There's no mentioning of safety. There's mentioning only of how to achieve respect—that's a big difference. Mostly people speak only of the need for safety, "Oh, we have to protect the other patients", even if it doesn't make any sense. They entertain the worst case scenario, "something bad could happen". And so they're cracking down on a scared person and you get a logic of fear amplifying itself—the patient's logic of fear and the staffs' logic of fear feed off of each other.

The other thing I'm frequently up against is that staff will put someone in restraints before I even get to the unit. So I actually don't even have a choice because the choice has already been made. Sometimes I have sat down with staff after an incident and asked people why they thought it was necessary to put the patient in restraints and how they got to that conclusion. And usually, to staff, that question feels like I'm not protecting the safety of the staff. So there's a lot of anger and fear that arises between the nurses and me. Often the idea that the use of restraints could be traumatizing for the patient is not considered either. What is considered is only the safety of staff—so then it follows that you can do whatever it takes to maintain 'safety'.

Staff will then talk to the person who is in restraints as if they could hear and understand what is being said, which, again, denies what we know from behavioural science. When someone is terrified, words don't really have a big effect on them. And, when someone's terrified, they're responding with a logic of fear and terror, which may be more gestural than verbal and they won't likely be calm and thoughtful and able to reason. So to say this person is being defiant is a *reading into* their behaviour as opposed to understanding that 'this is a person who is in restraints now and is afraid and he probably feels indignity'.

The feeling of indignity is probably intensifying the person's fear because now that the boundaries of his own body and safety have been overcome by other people's needs, so what's next?

Editorial Note:

Dr. Belnap's question on behalf of the patient "so what's next?" raises the larger question of 'how far will the other go?' Or, in other words, the overcoming of a person's boundaries and sense of safety raises the question 'If I can be put in restraints and given medication without my consent, is there really any limit to what the other can do to me?!'

BB:

So you've got a patient who's terrified and you've got staff talking as if this person could reason, which is a big mis-attunement, and this may be re-traumatizing. That is the ordinary scenario. Then there is often an immediate request to me, the psychiatrist, from staff—"This person's out of control and they need medication"—which is a *chemical* restraint. The Department of Mental Health in Massachusetts has been doing a lot of training to change how restraints are used. The training has been focused on the idea that, although they may sometimes be necessary, we have a responsibility to patients to minimize the number of restraints, and to recognize that restraints are traumatizing and are potentially harmful to patients. I see a lot less restraints being used now that there are people working much harder to make a link to the concerns of the patient and to give the concerns and worries of the patient a place to be heard.

BF:

Now, you are speaking of both chemical (medication) and physical restraints. Can you elaborate on the relationship between the two types of restraints?

BB:

Usually physical restraints are used first. Chemical restraints come in when someone is in an agitated state and the nurses feel and believe that this person is going to stay in an agitated state if they don't get medications. Often the patient has been refusing medications and they don't have a Rogers order yet.[4] However, in my experience, the truth is that both types of restraints may come about because of an effort to have an authority recognized by a psychotic person. It is often assumed that the person in psychosis 'isn't following the rules', and then there is a stand-off between staff and patient. Then limit setting may be[] practised as 'holding a harsh limit' and speaking aggressively to the patient about the need for limits on the unit, as in, "this is just what you have to do". This approach conveys a threatening tone towards the patient.

If the patient doesn't respond in the desired way to limit setting then they're considered 'defiant'. If a patient is defiant, 'safety' may then be interpreted to require that the patient submit to, or recognize, the rules of the unit—this can lead to a stand-off that gets aggressive. What I often notice is that the expression of aggression by the psychotic person can very quickly be read by staff as impending violence. And then the staff often reacts pre-emptively in a way that is fear-based which, in itself, is often provocative.

Furthermore, there's often an indignity that precedes the patient becoming upset and that precedes the patient being restrained. For example, there is usually a particular difficulty that arises for the patient. Let's

[4] In this instance the term "Rogers order" refers to a type of guardianship (Rogers Guardianship), active in the state of Massachusetts, where a person's guardian has been granted the authority by the court to allow the administration of antipsychotic medication without the patient's consent.

say the patient is being restricted from going to the kitchen or restricted from making a phone call. And the patient then says: “Wait, I have rights. I have [a] right to go to the kitchen. I have a right to make a phone call.” And then the staff assumes a rigid position such as “No, these are the rules of the unit”. Imagine the alternative in which, rather than having a struggle between staff and patient over ‘rules versus rights’, perhaps there could instead be another type of conversation where the patient can be allowed their dignity in trying to grapple with the disappointment and difficulty inherent in being in a place [hospital] where he feels that his rights are being infringed upon.

Perhaps the patient is saying he’s “king of the universe” or he has a “special relationship with Obama”. His claim that he has a “special relationship” to people in power has truth to it. What if that kind of statement could be heard more often by the nurse or mental healthcare worker as metaphorical and as a strategy by the patient to make himself feel like he is someone who has dignity? And the patient, in this example, does in fact have a relationship to people in power. Ideally we all do, right? Ideally, power links all of us to a place where our rights are protected. Ideally, power is a kind of relationship where, as an individual, the law protects us from indignities based upon our basic rights that we assume secure our sense of humanity and sense of safety in the world. We suppose that our security and safety are being protected by the people who represent the law.

We need to have these types of complex conversations that address the relationship between the rules of the unit and the patient’s sense of dignity, their safety in the world and their sense that there is a social order that has them in mind as an individual, and is protecting their comfort and their rights and their access to things. A space is needed for that type of conversation and I don’t think that space is built into the culture of most hospital units. Instead, we go quickly to fear and managing the safety of the other patients. For example, we often say: “This patient’s loudness is bothering other patients … we have to subdue them because of our responsibility to other patients … this patient is frightening other patients.” Instead, we should be saying: “If he is frightened, how do we care for the other patients *and* this one?” So these are the real, more common, everyday difficulties on the inpatient unit.

There is safety that comes through understanding and there is safety that comes through control. The safety that comes through control is different than the safety that comes through understanding and real listening. Communicating with an open face, just speaking and trying to understand is stabilizing to the person who is experiencing psychosis. And I think that this stance of 'wanting to understand' is stabilizing to everyone else who witnesses it because you're watching sense and meaning being made. There is actually more stability in working together to make sense of something that links us all than there is [in] attempting to impose control over someone. Because I think that when you do the latter, there's always the question of where is that line? Where are you going to draw it on me? How much anger can I express before you say no?

I think that how you interpret safety 'risk' has a lot to do with your idea about what safety is. Again, with regard [to] my example of the hospital unit, when I walked down to the unit I didn't see any safety risk. I don't think the other patients did either, partly because the mental health worker wasn't afraid of herself or the parts of herself that were similar to the patient. Also, she wasn't afraid that by making a connection to this patient, other people would judge her if they perceived her to not be following protocol.

BF:

Well, in your way of speaking about it, can we say that fear often precedes the safety risk? As you said, you went on the unit and you didn't see a safety risk. And the reason you think that was the case is because she, the mental health worker, wasn't afraid. That is an interesting reversal. We typically think that because there's a safety risk, one becomes fearful.

BB:

Right. She wasn't afraid and nor was the other staff member standing by her side. Nor were the other children who were on the unit because there was a relationship that was taking place, they [patient and worker] were talking about the problem, and they were going to transition to another space. I think there was a process being witnessed. Other patients on the unit felt safe when they saw people who were very engaged with a calming tone of voice or a voice that's really trying to make a connection. So I think that is, partly, an answer to your question. She, the mental health worker, wasn't afraid, but more than not being afraid she was interested. She was curious. She was available. She was looking into herself and inside of him and they were talking about a range of things that were important to them.

So there were things to be afraid of that could be talked about and they were put in a context. She said she understood why the patient would be mad and upset and angry or maybe even afraid of those people outside the door. Dr. Les Havens, from Cambridge Hospital in Massachusetts, would do the same thing. When a psychotic patient was fearful and upset, he would say: "Oh yes, there's so many reasons to be afraid." And he would take it to the *n*th degree where the psychotic patient would often say: "Dr. Havens, it's okay. Things can get that bad, but they're not that bad now!" And, because he told the truth by saying "Yes. People can be awful, terrible", fear was given a place in a bigger story. Fear is our human connection. It's not the thing in you that I have to protect myself from.

8.2.1 Discussion: Our Common Vulnerability Under the Law or, "Fear Is Our Human Connection … Not the Thing in You That I Have to Protect Myself From"

Dr. Belnap's formulation of fear as "our human connection" gives us a way to consider fear as a common ground upon which to build a relationship with someone experiencing psychosis. As Dr. Belnap emphasized, the key element that allowed the mental health worker's intervention to succeed was her capacity to use her own history of extreme experiences to better understand the experience of the patient. She noted: "Because of her cultural experience she had no trouble sharing parts of herself with the patient—she was not afraid or ashamed." Furthermore, similar to Dr. Havens, the mental health worker could acknowledge that "yes, there is a lot to be afraid of", and thus she transformed fear from something to be avoided into a source of connection and understanding. Thus Dr. Belnap arrives at the conclusion that fear "is not the thing in you that I have to protect myself from". Fear is to be expected and it makes sense.

Dr. Belnap's discussion of how authority might be understood and exercised on the inpatient unit is very important for our understanding of how to approach someone who feels misheard and misunderstood, and is in distress. As Dr. Belnap notes in our discussion, "[t]he truth is that some of these restraints [physical and chemical] come about because of an effort to have an authority recognized by the psychotic person". I suggest that there are also verbal strategies (verbal 'restraints') that clinicians and staff use in an effort to *psychologically* subdue a patient who may be expressing their fear through extreme ideas, the content of voices, and gestures. For example, clinicians will often respond to a person expressing distressing beliefs ('delusions') either with 'reality testing' techniques or by directly challenging the veracity of the person's beliefs. Rather than create a space to understand the value and meaning of a person's distressing beliefs and voices clinicians typically move quickly towards urging the person in psychosis to recognize the authority of consensual reality.

In the course of the interview, Dr. Belnap discusses two versions of how authority can be represented by staff. First, she discusses a version of authority that is rigid and is deployed to compel patients to conform to certain rules and regulations. Dr. Belnap's most poignant example of this type of authority is evident in her discussion of how hospital staff sometimes tends to emphasize safety over respect. Dr. Belnap suggests that the rigid form of authority arises out of fear and aims to maintain control. Most importantly, the rigid form of authority tends to compound and amplify the patient's fear. Dr. Belnap observed that "when [hospital staff] … entertain the worst case scenario … they crack down on a scared person and you get a logic of fear amplifying itself—the patient's logic of fear and the staff's logic of fear feed off of each other". In the course of my discussion with Dr. Belnap a new insight emerged regarding the relationship between fear and safety. Typically, we assume that a safety risk—a presence of danger or violence—precipitates fear. In Dr. Belnap's exploration of how fear can function on the hospital unit it is clear that fear can very well precipitate the onset of *perceived* unsafety, thus leading staff to resort to harsh measures to restore safety. With regard to the patient in Dr. Belnap's example, although the patient on the unit was initially quite agitated, yelling and banging on the door, Dr. Belnap observed that the other people on the unit were not in a state of heightened fear. The single patient's outburst did not create a climate of fear amongst the other residents on the unit. Dr. Belnap explained that, "[o]ther patients on the unit felt safe when they saw people who were very engaged with a calming tone of voice or a voice that's really trying to make a connection". The patient was not approached with fear, but instead with understanding, and therefore a sense of containment and safety was preserved on the unit. Dr. Belnap noted that the mental health worker was not afraid but in addition to being unafraid, "[s]he was curious and she was available. She was looking into herself and inside of him and they were talking about a range of things that were important to them".

Understanding—versus attempts to control—is more likely to create a sense of safety and 'stability'.

As an alternative to the rigid form of authority, Dr. Belnap introduced a version of authority that is utilized to protect the person in psychosis from fear-driven, and often harsh, limit-setting measures. The latter version of authority would allow the person experiencing psychosis to speak about and process their ambivalent experience of authority (or the limit) *itself*. For example, as Dr. Belnap notes in our earlier conversation,

> [r]ather than having a struggle between staff and patient over 'rules versus rights', perhaps there could instead be another type of conversation where the patient can be allowed their dignity in trying to grapple with the disappointment and difficulty inherent in being in a place [a hospital] where he feels that his rights are being infringed upon. (p. 192, Chap. 8 of this text)

In order to avoid making the error of relying upon a rigid and purely disciplinary version of authority, the representatives of authority must be careful not to align themselves, in total, with the limit itself. Both patients and staff must be allowed to acknowledge the potentially harsh application of rules and limits. Alternatively, patients and staff must be allowed to speak about the fact that rules and limits, and the 'Law' itself, are fundamentally flawed and may indeed fail to protect. Dr. Belnap highlights this latter point when citing the message that Dr. Havens would often express to patients in distress: "Oh yes, there's so many reasons to be afraid." I read Dr. Havens' intervention as at attempt to acknowledge the fact of our universal vulnerability under the Law, such that the Law, and its applications, via various symbolic limits and rules, can indeed fail to protect.

With the rigid use of authority the patient's resistance to rules is viewed by staff as a defiance of authority and thus triggers a severe response by those who represent the authority. In the alternative, and dignifying, use of authority the representative of authority assumes a stance of curiosity about the patient's 'defiance' and assumes that the purpose of the patient's defiance has value and can be understood. With regard to a patient's claim of "having a special relationship to Obama" or of being "king of the universe", Dr. Belnap asks:

> What if that kind of statement ["I'm king of the universe"] could be heard more often by a nurse or mental healthcare worker as metaphorical and as a strategy by the patient to make him feel like he is someone who has dignity? And the patient, in this example, does in fact have a relationship to people in power. Ideally we all do, right? Ideally power links all of us to a place where our rights are protected. Ideally, it is a kind of relationship where, as an individual, the law protects us from indignities based upon our basic rights that we assume secure our sense of humanity and sense of safety in the world. We suppose that our security and safety are being protected by the people who represent the law. (p. 192, Chap. 8 of this text)

In their co-authored book chapter in *The Austen Riggs Reader* titled "What Is Psychodynamic Psychopharmacology? An Approach to Pharmacologic Treatment Resistance" (2011), Dr. Belnap and Dr.Mintz discuss how a patient's resistance, non-compliance, and defiance can be unpacked and understood if the clinician has the patience and curiosity to explore the purpose of the non-compliance along with the patient.

In the following excerpt Dr. Belnap and Dr. Mintz discuss the case of a woman who was diagnosed with "schizophrenia" and who "could only tolerate antipsychotics [medication] that were ineffective" (p. 46). The following example is useful in helping us understand how to find the subjective meanings that underlie a patient's resistance, whether the object of resistance is a medication regimen or particular rules within a treatment setting:

> For example, consider Ms. A, who sought help at her family's urging for treatment refractory schizophrenia. She had previously been able to organize herself enough to competently raise a child with support from her parents. After her son's death from cancer, she could only tolerate antipsychotics that were ineffective. Invariably, when considering a switch to more effective medications, she became frightened of becoming depressed and killing herself. Her preoccupation with the hallucinated voice of her dead child and delusional conviction that she could bring back the dead revealed the powerful logic behind her treatment resistance. If she became non-psychotic, then her child was forever lost; she feared that the grief of this loss would kill her. She unconsciously resisted effective treatment because improved reality testing could interfere with restitutive psychotic efforts (Havens, 1968; Nevins, 1977), with the potential to precipitate a grief reaction that could overwhelm her already limited capacities and risk suicidal depression. (Belnap and Mintz, p. 46)

This passage appears in the chapter under the subheading "Remember that symptoms are not only problems—they are also solutions" (p. 46). In the case of Mrs. A, as the authors suggest, the patient's psychosis (her symptoms) served the purpose of protecting her from the overwhelming grief of losing her child. Her 'resistance' to an effective medication regimen could have very easily been read by her providers as 'non-compliance' and as an act in defiance of 'best practices'. Fortunately her providers did not accept her resistance at face value but instead were curious and able to help the patient discover the "powerful logic behind her treatment resistance". As the author's note, Mrs. A "needed to see how her psychosis deepened her loneliness before she was able to change and accept more effective anti-psychotic medications" (Belnap and Mintz, p. 59).

At this juncture we might ask how the patient's use, and experience of, the 'effective' (versus 'ineffective') medication could differ without her 'resistance' and her subsequent discovery of the logic behind her resistance. In other words, would an initial passive acceptance of effective medication have precluded her from facing the underlying grief? As Belnap and Mintz note elsewhere in the same chapter, "[w]hen medications signify that a patient has symptoms *rather than feelings*, meaningful opportunities for self-understanding can be lost" (italics added, Belnap and Mintz, p. 49). Herein lies the significance of Belnap and Mintz's term "psychodynamic psychopharmacology". Without careful attention to the psychodynamics that underlie the patient's ambivalent relation to medication, we run the risk of losing the knowledge ("self-understanding") contained in the patient's resistance.

In the same fashion we can view Dr. Belnap's anecdote regarding the patient who claims to have "a special relationship with Obama" or who likewise claims to be "king of the universe" through the lens of curiosity. Rather than dismiss such statements as 'delusional and grandiose', which would only serve to pathologize and likely shut down the patient's speech, Dr. Belnap argues that we should make an effort to understand the patient's claims to power as a "strategy by the patient to make him feel like he is someone who has dignity". When we categorize statements such as "I'm king of the universe" or "I've been chosen to become a Nobel Laureate" as either non-sensical or even as simply grandiose we run the risk of finding ourselves in opposition to the patient and in a struggle over the nature of reality. If we instead begin with the premise that such statements and claims are metaphorical then we will more likely find ourselves in a position of 'ally' and 'co-researcher' with the patient and with the shared goal of discovering the meaning and significance of the person's speech and behaviour.

References

Apollon, et. al. (2002). *After Lacan: Clinical practice and the subject of the unconscious.* (Eds.), R. Hughes & K.R. Malone New York: SUNY Press.

Belnap, B., & Mintz, D. (2011). What is psychodynamic psychopharmacology: An approach to pharmacological treatment resistance? In E. Plakun (Ed.), *Treatment resistance and patient authority: The Austin Riggs reader* (pp. 42–65). W.W. Norton & Company.

Davoine, F., & Gaudilliere, J. M. (2004). *History beyond trauma*. Other Press.

Gaudilliere, J. M. (2021). *Madness and the social link* (F. Davoine, Trans.). Routledge.

Rogers, A. (2016). *Incandescent alphabets: Psychosis and the enigma of language.* Karnac Books Ltd.

9

Bridging the Gap Between Psychotic and Non-Psychotic Experience

"When the inside and outside have been breached, it is only in between that it is possible for anything to be shown."
—Davoine and Gaudilliere, *History Beyond Trauma,* p. 59

9.1 Fear, and Transference Impasses: When Analytic Neutrality Does Not Work

This chapter will address the gap that too often derails the analytic relationship between the clinician and the person experiencing psychosis. Current misunderstandings of psychosis stem from biological reductionism[1] and, more fundamentally, from an underlying fear of psychosis. The

[1] Individuals experiencing psychosis are at risk of being misunderstood or of having their experience deemed incommunicable. It is not uncommon to hear within the fields of psychology and psychiatry that it is pointless or even dangerous to encourage people who experience psychosis to speak at any length about their inner experience of voices, messages, and disturbing beliefs. It is said that insight- (meaning-) oriented therapy, much less psychoanalysis, is not appropriate for treating psychosis. In mainstream mental health settings, treatment for psychosis is typically symptom-oriented where medication management of symptoms is the mainstay combined with social services and perhaps supportive counselling. We do not hear much about the possibility of fundamental change for the person struggling with psychosis. By fundamental change I mean the transformation of

B. Fimiani, *Psychosis and Extreme States*, The Palgrave Lacan Series,
https://doi.org/10.1007/978-3-030-75440-2_9

interviews in Chaps. 7 and 8 with Cindy Marty Hadge and with Dr. Rogers and Dr. Belnap, respectively, have given us new insights into how fear pervades the experience of both users and providers of treatment services. The interviewees' responses also serve as a guide regarding how fear can and must be overcome in order to make connections with people experiencing psychosis.

As I have demonstrated in previous chapters, Lacanian psychoanalysis is a vitally important approach to working with people who experience psychosis and other extreme states. Lacan, like Freud, had a deep respect for the experience of, and the specific *knowledge* inherent to, psychosis. The clinical approach that I have laid out in this book provides us with a guide on how to understand, listen to, and intervene in psychosis in a way that can create the possibility of a symbolic treatment of delusion and voices. However, there is one caveat to my approach that remains to be addressed in order for clinicians to make the most effective and authentic connections with people experiencing psychosis. In previous chapters I have promoted an approach to handling the transference, and to occupying the position of the analyst, that hews quite closely to the orthodox psychoanalytic concepts of 'analytic neutrality', or what is sometimes termed the 'absence' of the analyst. However, with certain patients

---

one's relation to one's experience (and symptoms), rather than simply the suppression or control of symptoms. A main problem that we face is the biological reductionism within psychiatry and the influence biological psychiatry imposes over the mental health field. People with psychosis are still being advised by providers within the medical model that they have a progressive brain disease and that, if they are diagnosed with psychosis, they should not entertain ambitious goals like having a family or a productive career. Of course statements such as these are inaccurate and disheartening. Various effective psychological and social approaches are well documented, and there are countless personal narratives of recovery that illustrate how people who experience psychosis are living full lives.

I direct the reader to several resources, including books and organizations, that can illustrate alternatives to the biological-psychiatric reductive point of view of psychosis. First, Marius Romme, MD, and Sandra Escher, Ph.D. et al. have authored and edited several books that dispel the myth that people who experience psychosis are condemned to overall poor prognoses. Their books include *Living with Voices: 50 Stories of Recovery* (2009), *Psychosis as a Personal Crisis: An Experience Based Approach* (2012), and *Young People Hearing Voices: What You Need to Know and What You Can Do* (2010). Second, organizations including the *International Society for the Psychological and Social Approaches to Psychosis* and the various regional and national chapters of the *Hearing Voices Network* are of vital importance in contesting reductive approaches to psychosis and in generating awareness of progressive clinical and peer-driven approaches to understanding, treating, and recovering with psychosis. Furthermore, the testimonies documented in Chaps. 7 and 8 of this book by Cindy Marty Hadge and Dr. Annie Rogers respectively offer a strong rebuke to such low expectations.

experiencing psychosis I have found that a neutral stance within the transference can lead to a transference impasse where the patient may respond by explicitly ending the treatment (e.g. perhaps in anger following my refusal to meet a particular request) or, inexplicably, drift away from the treatment.

My analytic training taught me to maintain a stance of 'analytic neutrality', or absence, regardless of the patient's psychical structure. With regard to working in the field of neurosis, the fundamental guideline of analytic neutrality is rooted in Lacan's teaching on the topic of transference. In *Seminar XI*, Lacan (1978) discussed how the analyst's desire "remains an x" so that "the crossing of the plane of identification is possible" (p. 274). In other words, in the field of neurosis, the analyst's desire must remain an "*x*" or an 'unknown' (e.g., absent/neutral) in order for the subject to emerge from behind, or within, the discourse of the ego. Lacan explains that, driven by the analyst's absence, "[t]he experience of the subject is thus brought back to the plane at which, from the reality of the unconscious, the drive may be made present" (p. 274). In Chaps. 3 and 4 of this book I discussed at length what I termed the 'reversal' of the transference in the field of psychosis. My conception of the reversal of the transference, although in important ways radically different than transference in neurosis (i.e., in psychosis the analyst is not cast by the psychotic as a '*subject-supposed-to-know*'), still largely maintains the position of the analyst as neutral or absent.

The patient represented in the clinical example discussed in Chap. 6 responded seemingly very well to my position of absence and neutrality. In response to my desire-to-know (desire presented as an '*x*') the patient's productive dream-work emerged to challenge his delusional thought process, thus raising a new question that served to undermine the certainty of his delusion. I established that his internal question was both a response to the position of the analyst and evidence of the subject of the unconscious emerging from the confinement of delusion. But not all patients are receptive to this more or less orthodox positioning of the analyst. I have encountered patients that seem to call on the analyst for something different than a purely enigmatic desire. Nonetheless, until relatively recently, I have methodically drawn the line where the neurotic patient seems to demand any response from the analyst that might sustain the discourse of the ego. Similarly, with regard to psychosis, I have, historically, drawn the line where the patient calls for a response from the analyst that could sustain rather than challenge the structure of delusion. This latter point alludes to the problematic of "collusion" with delusion. The ethical guideline implicit in the dictate of analytic neutrality has, in many instances with patients, led me to an impasse where the working relationship simply broke down.

My motivation to explore the topic of 'fear' in this book originated from my personal experience of fearfulness when working with people experiencing psychosis and other extreme states. There have been numerous sources of fear in my encounters with patients, *and colleagues*. As Dr. Belnap discussed so eloquently in Chap. 8, fear circulates within systems and amongst individual providers of treatment. One fear that is common amongst clinicians is the fear that one may be perceived, by other clinicians, as deviating from the standard or orthodox approach.

First, I have experienced fearful (and dreadful) moments with people experiencing psychosis when the patient conveys particularly traumatic and horrifying experiences that in turn evoke strong feelings in me. The phenomena of fear and dread on the side of the clinician are often explained, in accord with Lacanian orthodoxy, as the clinician's *own* transference. Other schools of psychoanalysis (e.g., Object Relations or Relational psychoanalytic approaches) might explain such an experience of fear as 'counter-transference' or the result of projective identification. Mainstream psychological approaches may term the clinician's experience of fear and dread as resulting from 'vicarious' or 'secondary' trauma. I do not deny the truth or usefulness of the aforementioned claims to explain fear on the side of the clinician. However, I have indeed reached certain moments with patients that have caused me to question the Lacanian premise which holds that the clinician's experience of fear and dread can only indicate a much-needed trip 'back to the couch'.

Second, in my capacity as a clinician, I have experienced a different type of fear related to the pull towards a (perceived) transgression of the Lacanian dictate of analytic neutrality. There is a strictness to the Lacanian approach to training analysts that demands adherence, by the analyst, to particular ethical principles designed to support a fidelity to the 'real' and to ensure that the subject of the unconscious is privileged and provided with an opportunity to speak. The ethics of Lacanian psychoanalysis guards against any analyst–patient dynamic that could collapse the space of the unconscious by reducing the analytic relation to 'dual' relation. Thus, when called upon by people experiencing psychosis to acknowledge a shared 'truth', I found myself at odds with my training, which guards me against entertaining the idea that there could be a shared 'truth' between me and my patient.

The claim that (self-)disclosure is unethical is axiomatic in the Lacanian field. There are sound technical and ethical reasons for abstaining from self-disclosure that I have either implicitly or explicitly discussed in a previous section of this book. The term 'self-disclosure' typically refers to the disclosure of personal details of the analyst's feelings, personal experiences, and thoughts. Self-disclosure, when framed as hazardous and unethical, refers to an instance where the analyst burdens the patient with his or her personal 'problems'. The hazard of burdening the patient is the common cause for alarm with regard to the use of self-disclosure. While I of course agree that it is unethical to burden one's patient with one's own suffering, I argue that there is a form of disclosure by the analyst (not of the *self* per se) that is called for at certain moments in treatment with people experiencing psychosis and other extreme states.

I believe that there is a common ground, or 'shared truth' regarding 'groundlessness', between people who experience psychosis proper (e.g., voice hearing, distressing beliefs, visions) and so-called non-psychotic people. Thus there may be times when the analyst is called upon to disclose his or her knowledge of this 'common ground' in order to become a credible other for the patient. I will later explore this question of a 'common ground' in conceptual terms, and through an analysis of Davoine and Gaudilliere's clinical contributions, to illuminate the stakes of acting against the technical and ethical requirements of neutrality.

The acknowledgement of a 'shared truth' can take place internally (to the analyst) or could be an 'explicit' acknowledgement in the form of a disclosure to the patient by the analyst. My question is: does such an acknowledgement by the analyst constitute 'self'-disclosure or is it possible that, in the field of psychosis, another type of disclosure is called for—a disclosure or 'acknowledgement' of a shared experience of the defect in Language and the Law? My question here refers back to my formulation in Chap. 6 of this book of the horrifying truth of the moral Law that the subject of psychosis is acutely aware of.

9.2 Françoise Davoine and Jean-Max Gaudilliere: "Zones of Non-Existence", "Annulment", and a Shared Truth

Françoise Davoine and Jean-Max Gaudilliere's work in their groundbreaking book *History Beyond Trauma* (2004) provide us with a point of departure from Lacanian orthodoxy with regard to the dictate of analytic neutrality, and a new way to understand the common ground (e.g., "zones of non-existence")[2] between psychotic and non-psychotic experience. Several years ago I met Françoise Davoine[3] at a national conference of the International Society for the Psychological and Social Approaches to Psychosis (ISPS). The ISPS is an organization that takes 'psychosis and extreme states' as its focus rather than privileging any particular clinical approach, whether psychoanalytic, psychiatric, peer support model, or other. Although Davoine and Gaudilliere's background is in Lacanian psychoanalysis, I became aware of their joint work in a context outside of the psychoanalytic field. Furthermore, I found that very few of my Lacanian colleagues were aware of Davoine and Gaudilliere's contributions. Despite my long-standing interest in psychosis, I also was unaware of Davoine and Gaudilliere's work until just a few years ago. Perhaps the relative ignorance of Davoine and Gaudilliere's work stems from the fact that their approach constitutes an intervention in otherwise unquestioned concepts fundamental to Lacanian psychoanalysis, such as the dictate of analytic neutrality.

Davoine and Gaudilliere's innovation issues from the way in which they speak about certain death zones, or "zones of non-existence", that

[2] As noted in Chap. 8, Françoise Davoine and Jean-Max Gaudilliere adopted the concept of "zone of non-existence" from psychoanalyst Gaetano Benedetti (1920–2013). See Françoise Davoine and Jean-Max Gaudilliere's discussion and application of this concept in *History Beyond Trauma* (2004) and in *Madness and the Social Link* (2021).

[3] Françoise Davoine's husband, Jean-Max Gaudilliere, died in 2015.

inhabit the body of someone experiencing psychosis and extreme states. The "zones" of non-existence are understood to be a field that can envelope the analyst as well as the patient. The zones of non-existence may evoke an experience in the clinician of their ownmost zones of death, or death drive, which, if not attended to by the clinician, can lead to an impasse in the transference and repeat a pattern of disconnection and alienation. I will emphasize the work of Davoine and Gaudilliere to discuss ways that we can traverse the void that often separates psychotic and non-psychotic experience—a void that, if left unaddressed, can lead to a 'transference impasse'. The void is made of 'zones of non-existence' already well known to the person experiencing psychosis and that may evoke horror in the clinician.

I approach therapeutic work with people experiencing psychosis by first opening a space for connection and with an ear towards understanding the meaning of their experience *for them, not for me*. I see my role as an analyst, at least in part, as a guide in helping others make meaning out of their madness. I am working clinically with people whose voices are mainly "negative" or, in other words, abusive and controlling; and so my focus, therapeutically, is in this area of experience where the person is suffering and being bombarded by voices and thoughts that want to annihilate her. However, my aim is not simply to listen to and witness expressions of psychotic experiences, but also to provide a *way forward* (i.e., treatment) in order to transform destructiveness.

I begin with the concept that for the person experiencing psychosis, her system of disturbing beliefs (delusion) serves a purpose. Furthermore, the person experiencing psychosis has (*or produces*) a specific knowledge vis-à-vis delusion and, to begin the treatment, the analyst's desire must be guided by this specific knowledge in order to open a path for the clinician to enter the 'experience' or what Davoine and Gaudilliere call the patient's "zones of non-existence".

The clinician's fear of madness is one gap that separates psychotic from non-psychotic experience, and recognizing this fear may be the first step in bridging the gap. Davoine and Gaudilliere (2004) speak to this issue in a compelling way. The authors view psychoanalysis as key in our effort to make contact with madness but not without levelling an important critique of traditional Lacanian ways of conceptualizing the analytic relation.

Davoine and Gaudilliere propose a role for psychoanalysis in the following way:

> Psychoanalysis is, as it were, one of the pathways that madness has found in this century to make itself understood by us. Through the slowness, regularity, and rigour of its setup, it enables the analyst to come into contact with, and exist in, the patient's zones of nonexistence. (p. 12)

The authors establish "zones of non-existence" as, necessarily, zones or spaces common to the analyst and to the patient and to the psychotic and non-psychotic alike. But how, when the combination of fear and misguided clinical training conspire to stop us, can we enter into what the authors call the patient's "zones of non-existence"? The authors argue that we have to further challenge the dictate of 'analytic neutrality'. And, on the issue of neutrality, the authors discuss the "horror" encountered by the clinician in the face of "madness" and trauma. The authors explain that this 'horror'

> is not a fault affecting the objectivity of the observer but a threshold that must be crossed in order to make contact with a world that is otherwise unreachable. (p. 58)

"*It is not a fault affecting the objectivity of the observer.*" I take this to imply that when one experiences 'horror' in the face of psychosis, it is not to be attributed, necessarily, to the analyst's transference, i.e., 'counter-transference', or a mishandling of the transference. Rather the experience of horror, fear, or dread is the price one must pay to cross the threshold, and to gain access to an other's subjective world. The horror is universal, and it is shared, but the analyst has to have a desire to know and acknowledge the horror. The horror is both inside and outside for both non-psychotic and psychotic alike. Davoine and Gaudilliere's guidance on how to enter into "zones of non-existence' is essential to our ability as clinicians to enter into extreme experiences.

9.2.1 Clinical Discussion

The following case example offered by Davoine and Gaudilliere helps us further understand the challenge posed to psychoanalysis when working in the field of extreme states. In Chapter 2 of their book, the authors show us how the clinician can be called upon by their patient to speak of what is felt but not known, and how "feelings that are not conscious" can be nonetheless apparent on the face of the analyst:

> For Henry, the analyst's office was probably the last chance before hospitalization. He was subject to periodic fits of clastic rage during which he broke precious art objects belonging to his family. He had never taken medication, although his situation had gone on since he had left the university, in which he was brilliant, a few years earlier.
>
> For a very long time he found it hard to speak about his daily life and seemed to be in a permanent state of humiliation over unfortunate decisions and broken relationships. [...] Late in the afternoon one Friday, his tone of voice changed abruptly. "You're gray," he told the analyst pointblank. Surprised by this unusually direct and uncanny judgement, she said nothing. Several times he came back to this comment, "you're gray." The analyst said she was tired at the end of the week and, to herself, thought about some form of projection. Henry really had nothing more to say. He reluctantly filled the rest of his session with trivia and long silences.
>
> The following Tuesday, he had hardly sat down when he declared that this was their last meeting. ... [H]e thanked the analyst for her goodwill and her efforts; he no longer wished to impose upon them. When he was practically on the threshold, she managed to say, "Friday you saw something that I couldn't feel when you noticed that shadow on my face. That morning I had attended a burial of a friend, and by the afternoon I had completely forgotten it. But this erasure wasn't proof of my indifference. On the contrary, I'd been shocked that he was put in the ground without a word from anyone, without a proper ritual. I'd come away with my mind blank, empty. What you saw on my face was the color of an impression that was not so much repressed as cut off, impossible to put into an image or a word". (pp. 61–62)

We can clearly see how a blind or 'blank' spot in the analyst's experience can lead to an impasse in the transference. In this example the patient detected the impression of death on the analyst's face that the analyst was ignorant of herself. As the authors note, the patient urged the analyst to "produce a new concept" in order to take account of the impression on the analyst's face and to name the cause of the experience that threatened to end the analysis. Davoine and Gaudilliere offer a new concept, "cut-out impression", to account for a zone in psychical life where no word or image is given to an experience. There are various levels at which the phenomenon of the 'cut-out impression' is functioning in the authors' case example. In the moments that comprise the analytic sessions, both the patient and the analyst were living with unnamed and cut-out impressions of loss and trauma. With his family, Henry had lived through war, "revolutions, disasters, pillaging, and massacres. They survived, and even did so successfully, on condition that they did not look back" (p. 63). The details of Henry's trauma secondary to war and migration were unnamed and therefore, the authors note, "annulled" by those close to him. Henry was trained to survive by 'not looking back' and through a process of rendering moments of his experience annulled and therefore non-existent.

Similarly to Henry, the analyst in this case was burdened by the weight of a death that was not properly recognized, 'ritualized', or remembered. The analyst, like Henry, was also suffering from the persistence of a 'blank' spot. The loss and burial of the analyst's friend passed "without a word from anyone" and thus her experience was not linked by a word, gesture, or image to the other(s)—the loss was not inscribed within the social link. However, there it was, nonetheless, casting a shadow over the analyst's face.

Davoine and Gaudilliere observe that it is precisely "[t]his kind of erasure [annulment] that could drive him mad, to the point of unceremoniously destroying things in his family home" (p. 62). The analyst in Henry's case knew that he suffered from the annulled and broken parts of his experience. The analyst must also have known that Henry had had several others in his life who participated in annulling the details of his trauma. Thus, when Henry saw the cut-out impression 'casting a shadow' over his analyst's face, he named it, and in naming it he called upon his analyst to respond. The analyst faced an ethical choice under the pressure of Henry's powerful observation. Davoine and Gaudilliere note that

> [Henry] had forced the analyst to report such an episode, one that was haunting her face. As though she had worn a mask invisible to her own eyes. (p. 63)

It is important to notice the authors' choice of words here when they state that Henry "forced" the analyst to report an aspect of her experience. As the authors say later in the same chapter, following Henry's observation, the analyst revealed a piece of her "private life" seemingly in contrast to the psychoanalytic "rule of benevolent neutrality" (p. 64). I do not think that this term "forced" is at odds with the analyst's 'choice' in how to respond. Instead we could say that Henry's act, in a sense, 'force[d] the issue' of how (from what position) the analyst might respond to an intervention such as Henry's. Henry forced the analyst to make an ethical choice, but it was the analyst's choice, nonetheless.

In the case of Henry, the analyst's first choice was to adhere to the rule of 'analytic neutrality'. When Henry initially named the analyst's "gray face", the analyst, from a position of neutrality, deflected Henry's observation when she stated that she was "tired" and, internally, reflected on how the patient may be engaging in "projection". However, following her initial choice, the analyst realized that maintaining a position of neutrality in this case would have had potentially catastrophic consequences for the analysis and perhaps even for the life of the patient going forward.

> If she [analyst] had continued in a position of neutrality, he would have "broken" her as an incompetent who was interfering with his research into the traces of a vanished history. (p. 62)

Henry would have "broken" the analyst just as he was prone to breaking "precious art objects" that belonged to his family when in fits of rage, so that "something had to be said about the broken pieces of their former history" (p. 63). Henry's "research" extended beyond those directly related to his personal traumatic history to include his analyst. Henry's history of having his experience annulled made him highly skilled at detecting when this type of annulment was occurring in others. Thus Henry, as Davoine and Gaudilliere note, could detect the "funereal impression" on the analyst's face with "scientific acuity" (p. 63). Henry knew that something was being annulled in the analyst while the analyst remained ignorant of what was happening in herself.

Henry's declaration that he intended to abruptly end ("break") his analysis jarred the analyst into awareness of how her own experience of loss had been annulled. Not only did Henry give his analyst an opportunity to inscribe and thus reclaim her experience of loss, but his threat to end the analysis provided the analyst a second chance to sustain rather than interfere with Henry's "research" into madness. Henry was in search of an address for his unnamed experience and the analyst, by making an adjustment in her position, was able to help him begin to construct such an address. If the analyst had not managed to speak of the true reason for her 'gray face', "[t]his rupture between them would obviously have pushed him toward a state of aloneness periodically marked by fits of rage" (p. 63).

As I have noted earlier, the choice of the analyst to share in the impression of horror should not be considered simply as a "fault affecting the objectivity of the observer" (p. 58). In the case of Henry, the analyst's choice of sharing the reasons for the funereal impression on her face could easily be interpreted as contrary to the doctrine of "benevolent neutrality" that pervades Lacanian and other schools of psychoanalysis. Davoine and Gaudilliere acknowledge this when they say "The challenging of the analyst's professional ethos had resulted in a sort of confession" (p. 63). But confession of what exactly? What follows in this section of *History Beyond Trauma* indicates that what is *confessed*—if we must use that term—is a knowledge and experience of an 'impression'. The authors take issue with any interpretation of this type of analytic act as somehow burdening the patient by unethically unloading one's suffering onto the patient:

> One should not, of course, unload one's problems onto one's patients. Quite the contrary: what is being done is *unloading strange, uncanny impressions from them*. (authors' italics, p. 64)

Davoine and Gaudilliere are hinting at something very important when they refer to the "unloading" of the strange and uncanny "*from*" one's problems. The authors raise a question about the status of the "so-called private life" of the analyst in a case such as Henry's. Indeed, Henry's analyst revealed an anecdote from her recent and problematic experience of loss when she shared the difficult circumstances of her friend's burial. Many analysts might dismiss such a decision as 'self-disclosure' and thus a violation of the neutrality typically understood to be essential to a successful handling of transference.

However, rather than debate the merits of the disclosure of private life, the authors take issue with the category of "private life" itself as indicated when they state "what does 'private life' mean in such a case" (p. 64). The "unloading *from*" indicates an extraction of the universal from the specific. In other words, when Henry's analyst chooses to speak of her experience of the burial, she is also speaking about the universal strangeness of encountering loss-without-words. The analyst speaks of her encounter with a hole, with annulment, where words and recognition for the loss should have been. The analyst's sharing of her experience of annulment and erasure serves as an offering to Henry. What does the offering consist of? First, by speaking of her experience, the analyst is able to offer herself as an ally to Henry and to therefore prevent a repetition where Henry surely would have, once again, witnessed the failure to symbolize loss and thus witness the erasure of the subject. The analyst's offer in this case certainly preserved the analysis and may have saved Henry's life. As Davoine and Gaudilliere conclude: "If the analyst had remained silent, the psychoanalytic work would have simply stopped there. Or worse" (p. 64). Of course the analyst was not entirely 'silent', even initially, when she told Henry that she was "tired" in order to account for her 'gray face'. What the authors are emphasizing here is that the analyst could not remain silent regarding the key underlying point that Henry forced upon his analyst—namely, that there can be large swaths of traumatic experience that remain unnamed and that thus persist and make one sick, or "mad".

We are approaching an important distinction that can free us from the debate about whether or not it is ethical for the analyst to 'disclose' aspects of her 'private' experience. Both Henry and his analyst have intimate knowledge of the experience of 'unnamed' encounters with loss. Again, as clinicians, we clearly do not want to burden patients with our personal problems. However, in clinical situations like Henry's the analyst may be called upon to speak about his or her strange and uncanny experience of the 'unnamed'. Henry's declaration that he had decided to leave his analysis presented a dilemma to his analyst. The minor aspect of the analyst's dilemma was the question of whether or not to break the rule of 'neutrality' and speak of her traumatic encounter with an unrepresented loss. The major aspect of the dilemma concerned the question of how, or if, the analyst could come to terms with the object casting a shadow over her face. Henry was calling upon his analyst to provide him with a reason to trust her. Would his analyst maintain the pretence that she was just "tired" or would she speak of the 'horror' of encountering the annulment of loss?

Henry's history was littered with others who had failed to inscribe the losses and traumas of his life. Would his analyst provide him with an O/other, an address, capable of receiving and recognizing the existence of his losses? Could his analyst risk the "horror" at stake in entering into what Davoine and Gaudilliere call the "zone of non-existence" created in Henry's experience by the series of annulments?

There is an implicit question in Henry's observation of his analyst's countenance ("you're gray"). As Davoine and Gaudilliere acknowledge, Henry's analyst "had worn a mask invisible to her own eyes", but Henry had nonetheless "received a funereal impression" (p. 63). Henry named the analyst's "gray" mask. Henry was concerned more with the mask *itself* than with what was being hidden by the mask. Henry's implicit question to his analyst then may be formulated as 'what do you know about the experience of annulment and of having your experience of loss muted?' The analyst's initial response to Henry's implicit question was to deny that anything had been erased or annulled, which in turn caused Henry to declare that he was ending his analysis. It was the analyst's denial (continuing to wear her mask) that was, we can now see, the object of Henry's anger and 'horror'. *The horror in question regards the 'annulment' of loss, not simply the loss itself.*

Davoine and Gaudilliere's subtitle for the section of their book in which the case of Henry appears is "Casus Belli in Analysis" (p. 61). The 'casus belli' or 'just cause' for Henry's decision to end his analysis was the analyst's initial failure to acknowledge the fact that her own experience of loss had been annulled. Under the pressure of Henry's just cause to end the analysis, the analyst was moved to acknowledge the truth of what happened at her friend's burial. Were Henry and his analyst in a similar position with regard to the failure of the Other, and of language, to register their respective traumas? In Henry's case, the analyst succeeded in meeting the patient on a common ground and she succeeded in acknowledging a shared truth—a truth common to all subjects and a truth that corresponds to an encounter with death and the insufficiency of language to fully inscribe it. In essence, the analyst's words and actions communicated that '*yes I too know something about the defect in language and in the universe*'. With her choice to disclose her experience of the trauma of language the analyst established a credible address—a credible other—for Henry. Therefore the analysis, and thus Henry's 'research' in the field of madness and trauma, was allowed to continue.

9.3 Co-creating a Credible Address for the Treatment of Psychosis

In psychosis and extreme states, the Other as guarantor of a limit, and as a site of inscription, has been rendered incredible by certain internal and/or external catastrophic events. In Chapter 1 of *History Beyond Trauma* (2004), Davoine and Gaudilliere discuss how the 'Other of speech' has failed to inscribe the 'catastrophe':

> The imminent catastrophe ... has already happened but could not be inscribed in the past as past, since in this respect the subject of speech was not there. Nothing in the other was given him, no speech to name what happened there. [...] [T]he truth was unable to be transmitted. The information has remained a dead letter, outside the field of speech. (pp. 28–29)

How does the clinician operate in a space where Language has failed and where all symbolic limits have been ruptured (or perhaps never installed) so that the person experiencing psychosis is made vulnerable to voices and thoughts that are set free to say and do anything to the subject? Davoine and Gaudilliere ask: "How, then, to approach these regions [zones of death] where our patients have been and toward which they are, paradoxically, seeking to guide us?" (p. 29). The authors cite the following words of Lacan to further clarify the importance of the field of speech in creating a credible Other that could receive and inscribe (i.e., remember or historicize) the subject's experience of the 'catastrophe', trauma, or rupture. The authors cite Lacan (1977) from the "Function and Field of Speech and Language in Psychoanalysis" where he says:

> What I seek in speech is the response of the other. What constitutes me as subject is my question. In order to be recognized by the other, I utter what was only in view of what will be. In order to find him, I call him by a name that he *must assume or refuse* in order to reply to me. … Speech is in fact a gift of language. (italics mine, Lacan 1953, p. 86)

Psychotic speech, or speech that evokes an extreme experience, opens the possibility of an exchange, and the offer of speech posits an Other that can, as Lacan says, "assume" the position of listener or "refuse" to do so.

9.3.1 Clinical Discussion

Davoine and Gaudilliere offer a fragment of a case that sounds as though it was particularly challenging and perhaps, to some readers, may seem especially hopeless. The authors describe a moment in the case of "Gilda" where the patient seemed to emerge from her more typical state of all-consuming "madness" to address her analyst with words that convey great clarity about a shift, however momentary, in her relation to her madness. The authors explain that "one day, after fifteen years of madness and periodic hospital admissions, Gilda said to her analyst":

> Now I'm entering time. … Before I was running after time; I lived in non-time. I had no rest, never. I kept on running endlessly in the streets. The world of madness was flat. Everything was in black and white. I never stopped thinking. My only consistency was cogitation. Words ran on

> without stopping, while I remained, flat, behind the windowpane. Cut-off, with no contact with the world. (pp. 29–30)

In this passage Gilda conveys her experience prior to "entering time" where there was no other to hear and receive her experience, thus leaving her "behind the windowpane", radically alone. Her "entering time" seems to allude to the appearance of an other—her analyst we will discover—who was able to respond to her in a way that could inscribe her experience in time and put a stop to the incessant 'thinking" and, it is revealed, self-abuse. Gilda continues, further elaborating the details of her madness:

> Really I was the goddess: Isis, Kali, Lilith. I was the devil, the fallen angel Lucifer. Let no one say that this experience was nothing. [...] And I drank, to stimulate myself. I was a zombie. ... In the streets, so little of me was left. In fact, there was no me anymore. Only my wanderings across the ages. I was the Great Mother, the earth, ready to kill her creation, this humanity condemned forever. (p. 30)

Gilda then suggests how her analyst, by occupying a certain position, helped guide her "out of the hell of the streets":

> Now I realize that this [presumably the analysis] was like a journey. Like Dante's with Virgil, if that doesn't sound too pompous. Since I've known you ... [i]n fact, our six years were a journey into and out of the hell of the streets, of madness, of alcohol, and medications. After having said yes to me, one day you said 'no'. No to the streets, to the alcohol. I stopped everything, right away, including medications. Your 'no' wasn't a condemnation. Do you remember? (p. 30)

It was with the analyst's "yes" early in the case and, later, the analyst's "no" that a credible Other was created for Gilda.

In a discussion of Gilda's case earlier in their book the authors highlight the power of the analyst's "yes". Gilda says to her analyst: "Right at the beginning [of the analysis], you told me, 'Yes, it's possible to get out of madness'. You assured me that my craziness was a search, remember?" (p. 21). Davoine and Gaudilliere frame the work between analyst and patient as a joint 'search', or 'research', and delusion (madness) is understood as a "device" or 'engine' that drives the research rather than an illness or pathology to be eradicated. The authors cite historian of madness Jean-Marie Fritz (1992): "Madness is more a device than a destiny." Furthermore, madness is "a means of leaving the hell of misfortune, not the verdict condemning someone to an inexorable repetition" (Davoine and Gaudilliere, p. 23). The analyst's courageous statement that "yes", madness is indeed a form of research gave Gilda the hope she needed to find her way out of hell. It is clear from the account of the case that Gilda and her analyst came together around a joint research where madness and delusion served as the primary engine for their shared interest and pursuit. The authors note that "this process [analysis and co-research] was able to make use of the powerfully heuristic resources of delusion" (p. 22).[4] The analyst's offer of a joint effort to learn from madness and delusion created the conditions for credibility. In making such an offer to Gilda, the analyst conveyed that she 'believed' that Gilda's so-called delusion, and the processes underlying her delusion, constituted a research that could in turn produce knowledge about herself and about the 'social link'.

As the account of the case illustrates, Gilda perceived a 'no', a limit, from her analyst that, as she says, "wasn't a condemnation". The 'no', for Gilda, did not constitute a sign of disapproval or punishment by her analyst. Rather the analyst's 'no' served as an empty limit to Gilda's self-inflicted pain and suffering. Davoine and Gaudilliere continue: "The analyst had only a faint memory of this 'no', a no to the practices

---

[4] Upon meeting Gilda on the hospital ward, the analyst actually mistook her for a clinical "intern". The authors write: "Seeing her [Gilda] sitting there deep in conversation with a patient who declared herself to be the craziest on the ward, the analyst took her for an intern. 'Are you a psychologist?', the analyst asked, introducing herself as a psychoanalyst of the ward. 'No, I'm psychotic', she [Gilda] replied, smiling at the professional's confusion. 'I have frequent stays here'" (pp. 21–22). Davoine and Gaudilliere then elaborate on the emergence of the analyst–patient relationship defined as one of co-researchers: "[T]he analyst learned that Gilda had actually been a psychologist, and that her thesis had dealt with the 'streets of shame'." "She [Gilda] had entered her research, without affect, at the urging of a thesis director who was fascinated by the wretched of the earth and by the methods of participant observation. In this context, madness and the asylum were her only means of escape" (p. 22). Davoine and Gaudilliere continue: "Like all hospital inmates, who begin by ascertaining who they are dealing with, she [Gilda] asked, 'And you? What are you doing here?' 'I am an analyst, and also a researcher at the Ecole des Hautes Etudes en Sciences Sociales.' Gilda asked the analyst, 'What are you working on?' The analyst replied, 'Madness and the social link'" (p. 22).

stemming from ... lethal ideologies" (p. 30).[5] For Gilda, the analyst's 'no' was credible enough such that Gilda chose to stop pursuing, however temporarily, the 'lethal ideologies' driving her to be a "zombie" and to remain engaged with the belief that she was in turns a "goddess" and the "devil". In the course of the treatment, the 'no' seems to function only after the establishment, by the analyst, of the premise that states '*yes*, your madness has meaning, it is a form of research, and you [Gilda] can emerge from madness'. By joining together in co-research, Gilda and her analyst were able to establish a credible Other who could be the recipient and guardian of psychotic speech. Hope was established—hope, for Gilda, that she could live without her delusion and hope that she could stop destroying herself.

References

Davoine, F., & Gaudilliere, J. M. (2004). *History beyond trauma*. Other Press.

Escher, S., & Romme, M. (2010). *Young people hearing voices: What you need to know and what you can do*. PCCS Books.

Fritz, Jean-Marie. (1992). *Le Discours du fou au Moyen Age*. Presses Universitaires de France; Paris, France.

Lacan, J. (1977). The function and field of speech and language in psychoanalysis. In *Ecrits: A selection* (A. Sheridan, Trans.). W.W. Norton & Co.

Lacan, J. (1978). *The four fundamental concepts of psychoanalysis, the seminar of Jacques Lacan, Book XI* (J. A. Miller & Tr. A. Sheridan, Eds.). W.W. Norton & Co.

Romme, M., & Escher, S. (2012). *Psychosis as a personal crisis: An experienced-based approach*. Routledge.

Romme, M., Escher, S., et al. (2009). *Living with voices: 50 stories of recovery*. PCCS Books.

[5] My quotation here is truncated to capture only the essence of what is at stake in the interaction between the analyst and Gilda. However it may be of interest to the reader that the original quote is extended to include a reference to Pasolini's 1975 film *Salo* or *120 of Sodom* and to Visconti's 1969 film *The Damned* to emphasize the obscene and violent nature of Gilda's psychical life. The original quote reads: "The analyst had only a faint memory of this 'no', a no to the practices stemming from the lethal ideologies so frankly depicted in the films *Salo* (Pasolini 1975) and *The Damned* (Visconti 1969)" (p. 30).

Index[1]

[1] Note: Page numbers followed by 'n' refer to notes.

B. Fimiani, *Psychosis and Extreme States*, The Palgrave Lacan Series,
https://doi.org/10.1007/978-3-030-75440-2

Name Index[1]

A

B

C

D

F

G

[1] Note: Page numbers followed by 'n' refer to notes.

B. Fimiani, *Psychosis and Extreme States*, The Palgrave Lacan Series,
https://doi.org/10.1007/978-3-030-75440-2

Subject Index[1]

[1] Note: Page numbers followed by 'n' refer to notes.

B. Fimiani, *Psychosis and Extreme States*, The Palgrave Lacan Series,
https://doi.org/10.1007/978-3-030-75440-2

The manufacturer's authorised representative in the EU is Springer Nature Customer Service Centre GmbH, Europaplatz 3, 69115 Heidelberg, Germany. If you have any concerns regarding our products, please contact ProductSafety@springernature.com

Printed and bound by CPI Group (UK) Ltd, Croydon, CR0 4YY
30/09/2026
02225451-0005